Healing in Perspective

Healing in Perspective

Dewi Rees MD, FRCGP

Formerly Medical Director,
St Mary's Hospice, Birmingham,
and Senior Lecturer,
University of Birmingham

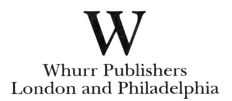

Whurr Publishers
London and Philadelphia

© 2003 Whurr Publishers Ltd
First published 2003
by Whurr Publishers Ltd
19b Compton Terrace
London N1 2UN England and
325 Chestnut Street, Philadelphia PA 19106 USA

British Library Cataloguing in Publication Data

A catalogue record for this book
is available from the British Library.

ISBN 1 86156 380 9

Typeset by Adrian McLaughlin, a@microguides.net
Printed and bound in the UK by Athenæum Press Limited, Gateshead, Tyne & Wear

Contents

Preface

I was standing in the ruins of Coventry Cathedral after the Litany of Reconciliation when I turned to the lady next to me and asked: 'How are you?' It was a conversational gambit, but she paused before she replied: 'I would normally say I'm all right, but as you are a doctor I will tell you how I really feel.' So I listened and she told me about her complaints and how she always felt physically better, and experienced less pain, after attending a church service. Later I learnt that, although her husband was a doctor, she took no medical treatment, being content to leave herself in 'the Lord's hands'.

Her firm belief that non-medical agencies could contribute significantly to her recovery did not surprise me, it is one that I have encountered on other occasions, but her words reminded me of the important part that a spiritual focus can play in the healing process. This needs to be recognized, nurtured and better understood, but the concept is already an essential part of many people's lives, as is evident from the large numbers who go on pilgrimages to Lourdes and other shrines, and who attend complementary therapists and spiritual healers. The Churches are also coming to terms with their dual commission to 'Preach the gospel and heal the sick' and many denominations now hold healing services – something that was a rarity forty years ago. Even more remarkably, I am told that in some Catholic churches complementary therapies are included in the healing mass.

With this burgeoning interest in healing, one thing is lacking: a sense of perspective. The subject raises so many questions. Is it effective? How does it work? How widespread is the practice? What happens on a pilgrimage to Lourdes and how will it affect a young person with an incurable disease? Who are these healers? What do they do? Is there any evidence to support their claims? This book considers such matters and tries to provide some of the answers.

Foreword

The Kingdom of God is the sum of right relationships.

These words of William Temple, Archbishop of Canterbury, in the 1940s, hold the clue to healing and wholeness, which is revealed, page by page, in this very special book, Healing in Perspective. If we have the right relationship with God, with family and friends, associates at work and in recreation, and with our own self, then we are likely to be a whole person. If our community, our council, our country have the right relationships with their counterparts, then we are well within sight of the kingdom that offers healing and wholeness, that gives meaning to life even if there is suffering in body, mind or spirit, or all three.

So I say 'Allelujah for this book', whose author, Dewi Rees (David to me and many other friends), sent me two chapters, after I had read the rest – chapter 1 about himself and chapter 9 'How is Healing Achieved?' The book is worth acquiring for these two chapters alone because, in them, we find Dr Rees has the balance, integrity and experience that reveal him as an example of all that we would like to achieve. He is the first to admit that he himself is nearer the completion of life in this world than many who will read the book, but he encourages all readers to explore their own path to healing and wholeness, contained in other chapters.

David is a Christian, as I am, but we both would always encourage those of other faiths and callings to follow their own way to healing and this book offers that opportunity.

David and I shared many services of prayer and healing in Coventry Cathedral. In my twelve years there, in a ministry that took me to many other countries as well, I came to realize the importance of four steps to healing:

- Penitence
- Forgiveness
- Reconciliation
- Healing

This happens at all levels from the individual to the international, where 'healing' could be called 'peace'. How often we saw it happen at those different levels.

I believe this book will be read world-wide, so I conclude by thanking David for all he has written and for honouring me by inviting me to write the Foreword. May your relationships and your wholeness be helped by it, perhaps even by what he says about this final word, offered in love: 'Shalom'.

John Petty
Dean Emeritus
Coventry Cathedral

Introduction

A great upsurge of interest in unconventional forms of treatment – both ancient Eastern and modern Western – marked the end of the twentieth century, and people now visit healers and alternative therapists almost as readily as they consult their family doctor. At the same time, complementary therapies are increasingly being offered in GP surgeries and hospital pain clinics, and there is evidence that doctors and healers are learning to collaborate more closely to provide optimum care for their patients. The medical establishment is responding positively to the changing market for health care and there are probably few medical schools that do not now offer courses in complementary medicine. In most instances these are optional, but in some countries they are compulsory. Politicians have taken note of these new trends and governments have been financing research in complementary and alternative medicine (CAM) since the early 1990s. In the United States funding is provided through the National Center for Complementary and Alternative Medicine (NC-CAM), a government agency which provided $69 million for CAM research in the year 2000.

The speed of this development has been dramatic. Many of the therapies are of recent origin: aromatherapy, the Bach Flower Remedies, LaStone therapy, the McTimoney technique, reflexology, Reiki and Shiatsu are all twentieth-century innovations, and some have even been devised by doctors. At the same time there has been a resurgence of interest in healing in the Christian Churches, often associated with a renewed zeal for evangelism. All this has had an effect on the way in which people view their illnesses and where they turn for help. But despite the vast number of popular books available on complementary medicine, there have been few, if any, attempts to place these therapies within their cultural and historical contexts. This book seeks to do just that.

Great care has been taken to avoid the use of jargon and to provide a book that is intellectually rigorous yet easy to read. Consequently, one possible point of contention has to be addressed. Should a distinction be made between 'being healed' and 'being cured'? Some people believe there is a difference and that it is important.[1] This problem does not arise in the French language as the word *guérir* is used for both 'to cure' and 'to heal'. I find this simple approach more helpful than one that emphasizes the difference between the words. In any case 'to cure' means 'to restore to health' and 'to make whole', which is what healing seeks to achieve. Indeed, in the preparation of this book I found so many definitions of the word 'healing' that I was reminded of the conversation between Humpty Dumpty and Alice in *Through the Looking Glass*:

> 'When I use a word,' Humpty Dumpty said in rather a scornful tone, 'it means just what I choose it to mean – neither more nor less.'

> 'The question is,' said Alice, 'whether you can make words mean different things.'[2]

When healing does occur it may be partial or complete, and people will often say that although they have not been completely cured they do feel better. An inner sense of well-being has been restored and this may be the result of a visit to a traditional healer or CAM therapist, or be the outcome of a pilgrimage or attending a healing service. These scenarios are all part of a healing spectrum that is a universal phenomenon and in this book we explore all these approaches, including the ancient urge to pilgrimage and the often unexpressed hope that the journey will result in the healing, not only of the soul but of the body too. We also look critically at the scientific evidence for healing and examine the way that healers of various traditions set about their task.

The book is intended for all those who are interested in healing in its many dimensions, but in particular for people who are actively involved in this field, whether as health care workers, clergy or complementary therapists. I have learned a great deal from practitioners who specialize in the more unconventional treatments and the need for such an interdisciplinary approach to the subject is becoming increasingly obvious.

The book contains case histories and, where appropriate, salient features have been altered to conceal the identity of individuals. The biblical references are included by permission of the New English Bible, Oxford University Press and Cambridge University Press 1961, 1970. Among the many people who have provided source materials and contributed in other ways I owe special thanks to Revd Tom Willis and Revd Aelwyn Roberts for their interest and help, and to the Very Revd Dr John F Petty, Emeritus Dean of Coventry Cathedral, for the gentle way he opened up the ministry of healing to me and for contributing the Foreword. Professor Brian Thorne has been closely involved in the book's development and I am very grateful for the many helpful comments he has made during the book's evolution.

Finally, and as always, I am most indebted to my wife, Valerie, who has cared for me for fifty years and has contributed so much to the writing of this book. It is dedicated to her.

Chapter One
Who is Dewi Rees?

It was suggested that I should begin with an account of my life so that readers might have an idea of what led me to write about healing. I was at first reluctant, believing that the work should stand on its own merits and be judged accordingly. But I realized that most books are produced by anonymous people whose lives and characters are hidden. Often this does not matter, but perhaps in this case it does. So this chapter is unashamedly autobiographical, offering the reader some insights into the development of my *Weltanschauung* which led to my commitment to holistic medicine and, ultimately, this book.

I was born in September 1929, of Welsh-speaking parents in the town of Barry, in South Wales. A doctor was present at the birth so there was a good chance that I was delivered by forceps. It was a pleasantly warm day. I was given the ancient Celtic name Dewi, but many people find it easier to call me by its English equivalent, David.

Barry was not the typical Welsh mining village, portrayed in books and films. It was a seaport, built for the explicit purpose of exporting coal, and never acquired the close communal spirit of the Welsh mining valleys. It was a time of great poverty with little work in the dockyards and with so many men on the dole that the schools were used as channels for the distribution of free meals, boots and milk to needy children. I attended Cadoxton elementary school. There were probably about 40 boys in my class, of whom two were black, which was most unusual in the UK in the 1930s. One of these boys was highly intelligent, the other not so, but neither received a higher education. The clever boy passed the 11+ examination for the county (grammar) school, but his father would not let him attend. Another boy and I also passed the exam: he went to the county school but left at the age of fourteen to become an apprentice to a painter and decorator.

My elder brother was a pupil at Llandovery College in West Wales and though my mother wished to keep me at home, I joined him there. This was during the Second World War and life was hard for everyone; most things were rationed and everyone was expected to work hard. This was certainly the expectation at Llandovery College. It was a small public school, with about 150 pupils and a great reputation for producing international rugby players and Oxbridge blues. It was also quite good academically and I have a photograph of myself in a 1st XV team which contained two future professors (Bristol and Cambridge) and a number of embryonic doctors, solicitors and school masters, though no clergymen. I liked the church services we had in the school chapel, and at the age of twelve I was christened and later confirmed into the Church in Wales.

After a compulsory spell of National Service in the army, I went to St Thomas's Hospital Medical School as a rugby player, but my heart was no longer in the game. I date this change in attitude to an incident that had occurred some years previously when, in a derby match with Christ College Brecon, the scrum collapsed and the Brecon hooker suffered a broken neck from which he later died.

In the same year, I was also greatly upset when the whole school were shown a newsreel that had been taken of the German concentration camps and became aware, for the first time, of the sufferings that had been endured in places like Belsen and Buchenwald. This made an indelible impression on my inner being and I still feel that the Holocaust was not just a Jewish experience, but one that is shared in varying degrees by people throughout the world.

The Pentecostal Tent

I first went to a healing service in 1947, the same year that I had my appendix removed in the Barry Accident Hospital. It was an emergency operation and I never discovered the identity of the surgeon who saved my life, but the event was probably instrumental in my deciding to become a doctor. I was the youngest patient on the ward: the bed to my right was occupied by a man whose leg had been amputated and who was quite talkative. An elderly man lay in the bed to my left; he was very quiet. In the morning his bed was empty and no one spoke about him afterwards. I realized eventually that he must have been very ill, that he had died during the night and that the nurses had taken his body to the morgue.

Following the operation, I was not allowed my normal sporting activities, which may explain why I wandered into the Pentecostal tent that had unexpectedly appeared on a bare plot of land on the outskirts of the town. During the late 1940s American evangelists, such as Oral Roberts, were undertaking 'crusades' in Europe, but at that time they were not making much impact in the UK. Wales had always been fervent for 'revival', but most people who attended church or chapel were distrustful of the Pentecostal movement, regarding it as too emotional.

Services in the tent were quite different from those I had previously attended, either at the Luchanna Mission — the small mission church for dock workers I attended with my father and where we sang Sankey and Moody hymns and listened to hellfire sermons — or in the almost empty Welsh Baptist chapel my mother favoured, or the Church in Wales services I attended at school. The Pentecostal services were lively, with cheerful songs and hand clapping, the music provided by a trumpet. I have fond memories of the elderly pastor, Mr Jones, who had served in the Welsh Guards before being converted, and of his daughter, Gwen, who was both welcoming and attractive. The chief crusader was a young man based in Cardiff: he was an extrovert with the gift of tongues, who tried to heal people with prayer and the laying on of hands. I cannot remember if he exorcized demonic spirits, but he probably did; it was that type of service. In retrospect it was like attending a lively out-patient clinic for the chronically sick, with the same people returning each week without showing much improvement.

Healing services are now so common in mainstream churches that it is difficult to appreciate that they were rare fifty years ago and the very idea of them unacceptable to most clergy and congregations. The fact that such services are now an important part of the religious scene is largely due to the enthusiasm for healing of minority groups such as the Pentecostal and Spiritualist Churches. It is interesting that the doctrinal approach of these churches is so different as some of their techniques are very similar. Both, for instance, favour the use of 'words of power'. One main difference is the emotional fervour of the Pentecostal service compared with the quiet approach of the Spiritualist service — at least in the UK; in other countries the pattern may be different.

Marriage

In 1952 I married Valerie, a Cardiff girl. We had met in London when we were both students but Valerie now had a degree in chemistry and worked in the laboratories at Hammersmith Hospital, whilst I was still an impecunious student. She helped to ensure that I passed my examinations, in particular that most boring of subjects, anatomy, which we learned to an excessive degree in those days.

1956 was an exceptional year for us: our first child, Eileen, was born in February and I passed my final examinations in April. Later, Eileen became the personal assistant to Peter Scott, the well-known painter and ornithologist, and is herself now a leading expert on water fowl. Anna, our second daughter, has a fulfilling life with her own family and also works full-time as a teacher of autistic children. David, the youngest, is the most individualistic of the three; he is a specialist in computer engineering.

Introduction to Spiritual Healing

When I married, I was given a book entitled *Divine Healing*.[1] It was a present from Marion Edwards of the South Wales Bible College, a theological college that had been established in 1936 in Vere Street, where I lived as a boy. The college was unabashedly evangelical and sought to train young men and women for any form of Christian work at home or abroad.[2] Its most famous alumnus is the Ulster politician, the Revd Ian Paisley. I remember him as well as the college principal, Mr Fidler, and his wife, but have no memory of Miss Edwards, yet her book is one of the few wedding presents that we still possess. I have never read *Divine Healing*, it is not my type of book, but I occasionally pick it up and glance at its pages, possibly expecting something to catch my eye. It was first published in 1934 and contains a personal testimony and a series of short meditations by the author, the Revd Andrew Murray. My copy is a fifth edition, so the book must have been quite popular.

In the preface, Murray offers the book as a testimony of his faith in divine healing, and goes on to say:

> After being stopped for more than two years in the exercise of my ministry, I was healed by the mercy of God in answer to the prayer of those who see in Him 'The Lord that healeth thee' (Ex. xv: 26). This healing, granted to faith, has been the source of rich spiritual blessing to me. I have clearly seen that the church possesses in Jesus, our Divine Saviour, an inestimable treasure, which she does not yet know how to appreciate . . . I can therefore no longer keep silence, and I publish here a series of meditations, with the view to showing, according to the word of God, that the prayer of faith (James v. 15) is the means appointed by God for the cure of the sick.

Whenever I read this preface I am struck by the author's sincerity. His book has too detailed a biblical exegesis for my taste, but I am sure that he had such a profound experience that he felt impelled to share it.

Junior Doctor

Early in my career I decided to become a General Practitioner, possibly because it was the path my elder brother had already taken. At that time there were no training schemes for GPs so I had to devise my own whilst, at the same time, ensuring the safety and welfare of my wife and baby daughter. I was fortunate in my parents-in-law, who were always ready to provide a home for us whenever the need arose, which was quite often. Valerie lived with them and took a Diploma in Education at Cardiff University, whilst I did my first resident hospital jobs in Bridgend and

Caerphilly. There I learnt the basic crafts required of a doctor, working first in medicine and then in obstetrics and gynaecology. The most junior doctors also had to work in the Accident and Emergency Department at nights and weekends, and all this provided a wider range of practical experience than would have been available in a teaching hospital.

The next year was spent in London as a trainee GP in a single-handed practice. The only training I received was during the first six weeks, as my trainer developed infectious hepatitis and had to retire to bed. By the time he had recovered I had become completely competent in managing the clinical side of the practice so he let me carry on and busied himself with other activities. I recognized that many of the people who came to me with physical complaints had underlying problems of anxiety or depression, but apart from listening and empathizing with their condition, had little to offer them therapeutically. However, diagnosing and treating iron deficiency anaemia was very rewarding at that time. It was a common problem in young married women and a course of iron tablets made an enormous difference to their ability to care for their families. Their anaemia was usually due to poor nutrition, heavy periods and multiple pregnancies. Contraceptive pills were not then available to control heavy periods and people no longer cooked in iron vessels, which previously had been a useful and reliable source of iron. Our ability to deal effectively with this widespread deficiency was due to a decision by the local hospital to provide GPs in its catchment area with open access to its pathology services. The hospital also provided the sterile syringes that enabled us to take and send blood samples to its laboratory. Then, because I wanted an opportunity to practise in a more demanding environment, we moved to Labrador.

Labrador

Sometimes known as the Land of Cain, Labrador is the poor relation of Canada, and though it lies within the same latitudes as the UK, the climate is much more hostile. There is an indigenous population of Inuit and North American Indians, as well as the descendants of settlers who emigrated from Europe in the nineteenth century. Life was very hard for these people, particularly before Dr Wilfred Grenfell visited the country in 1892. He was appalled by the health problems and poverty that he encountered and spent the rest of his life trying to alleviate them. His work was continued by the International Grenfell Association (IGA), a charitable body that provided medical and nursing services to the people of Labrador.

I joined the IGA as an assistant to Dr Tony Paddon at North West River and we moved to Labrador in 1958. Snow and ice covered the land for most of the year whilst mosquitoes and black flies were troublesome in the summer. The Inuit and most native Indians lived in wooden huts, though some of the Indians still preferred their tepees, even in the winter when the temperature would fall to −30°C. There was little work for them and they lived mainly on government handouts, supplemented by a little hunting and fishing. The Inuit always appeared cheerful whilst the Indians were invariably morose. Neither group appeared to have any recourse to traditional healing practices but relied entirely on Western medicine. Similarly, both had discarded their traditional belief systems and had converted to Christianity: the Indians to Roman Catholicism, while the Inuit joined the Moravian Church whose missionary input in that area dated from the eighteenth century.

North West River was an ethnically mixed community with a Hudson Bay store and a modern hospital run by Dr Paddon. He was supported by two English nursing sisters and a few aides, young untrained Inuit and Indian women who undertook basic nursing care and provided a translation service for patients who could not speak English. The area was rife with tuberculosis, but the worse of the epidemic had passed and the disease was being controlled by a combination of chest surgery undertaken in Newfoundland, and the new anti-TB drugs streptomycin, PAS and INAH. The IGA funded most of the medical care and patients received all treatment free of charge. The Newfoundland government covered the costs of two services: it paid for the TB programme and for an aeroplane (a Beaver) which enabled us to provide an air ambulance service for the patients and also to visit and hold clinics in outlying villages.

I arrived at North West River just in time to see the tail end of a diphtheria epidemic. I was taught to extract teeth as there was no dentist in the region, and I also learnt to take X-rays and provide a basic laboratory service for the hospital. Soon after we arrived Dr Paddon took his family on a much needed holiday and I was left in clinical charge of the hospital and a network of nursing stations which the IGA had established in the villages on the Labrador coast. In his absence I was expected to deal with situations which in the UK would be treated by experienced surgeons.

The first emergency involved a pregnant woman with a placenta praevia, a condition which could have led to the death of the mother and child. The diagnosis is not difficult, even without modern scanning techniques, and the management, involving a Caesarean section, is a routine procedure for skilled obstetricians, but the situation was very different for this particular patient. I had neither special training in surgery nor a proper theatre team. When we came to operate, the anaesthetic was given by a nurse who dripped ether onto a gauze mask which she held over the patient's face; my surgical assistant was a teenage Indian girl and we had no blood bank. Yet it was because of the recurrent vaginal bleeding that I felt forced to operate. I did a classical Caesarean section, the placenta was lying very low in the uterus and the baby and mother did well.

Other crises arose before Dr Paddon returned. These included having to deal with a hydatidiform mole, another serious complication of pregnancy, and with an Inuit fisherman who had a gunshot wound of the leg, which had become gangrenous. Although our plane was grounded by poor weather conditions, we were able to transfer him to St Anthony's Hospital in Newfoundland where the leg was amputated and he made a full recovery. Transportation south was masterminded by Jack Watts, a notable character in the community. He arranged for the patient to be taken to Newfoundland. However, to achieve this they had to transport him across two rivers in a row boat, then through a forest along a dirt track road on the back of a truck, before flying him some hundreds of miles to a landing strip where an ambulance conveyed him to the hospital. Some twenty years later, the same patient was readmitted to St Anthony's Hospital with a provisional diagnosis of peritonitis/appendicitis. He was found to have gas gangrene of the right psoas muscle, which was excised. Again, he made a complete recovery.

I find it interesting that during this period my religious beliefs tended towards agnosticism, but when I had to undertake operations that were beyond my clinical competence, I would send out 'arrow prayers' for help. This was an automatic reaction and not one that I had previously read or heard of. Yet in all the instances where I had need of such prayers the outcome was successful.

Learning Psychiatry

We returned to Cardiff after a year in Labrador, staying again with my parents-in-law. Not knowing what to do next, I went to see the medical director of the nearby Whitchurch (Psychiatric) Hospital and asked if I could go to the hospital and learn some psychiatry. He agreed and I spent a few days with one of the consultants, Dr Spillane, and then was offered the post of Senior House Officer, which I accepted. I am quite a good listener and everything seemed to go very well initially, then suddenly it all collapsed, not outwardly but inwardly. I became terrified and depressed. I was frightened that I would hurt other people or kill myself, but outwardly I continued to cope, knowing that I could not allow myself to crack. I had a discreet word with Dr Spillane, telling him as much as I considered appropriate, and he thought that my reactions augured well for my career in psychiatry as I was obviously a very sympathetic doctor. At night in bed I would shake from head to toe and Valerie would hold me in her arms and comfort me.

Then something happened that was pertinent to my mood. Two of my patients, both schizophrenic and, if I remember rightly, with first class university degrees, described themselves as being emotionally bankrupt. This touched a sensitive spot as that was precisely how I felt. Luckily, I had read some of Carl Jung's writings and I recalled him saying that the 'only cure for an affective disorder was conversion to a religion of light'. It also occurred to me that if you are emotionally bankrupt and need to recharge your inner batteries, you have to go to the source of love, which in my case was symbolized by Christ. So to the surprise of my family, I started to attend the local church, a practice I had not done since my teens when I had found it impossible to affirm the Christian Creed. So I went to St Mary's Church, Whitchurch where we had been married, and when the Creed was recited during evensong I remained silent. Then, over the months, I found that I could affirm the last part of this summary of the Christian doctrine and could say with increasing conviction that I believed in the communion of saints, the forgiveness of sins, the resurrection of the body and the life everlasting.

Slowly, over a long period of time and working backwards, I found that this declaration of Christian belief made sense to me and I was able to embrace it in a much more certain way than I had ever done before. But while I was resolving my inner turmoil I still had to support my patients and sometimes this was difficult. There were not many drugs available and electro-convulsive therapy (ECT) was still considered the best treatment for those who were severely depressed. To a large extent, ours was a 'listening therapy', but sometimes what we heard was hard to bear, particularly as I was going through 'a dark night of the soul' myself. I was helped by the *Don Camillo* books. Written by an Italian journalist, these works of fiction tell of the exploits of Don Camillo, a village priest, whose church houses a crucifix with which he converses. I found the use of a similar approach helpful. If any problem was too intense, I would visualize or think of the crucified Jesus and transfer the pain and guilt to him. The procedure worked well but I never realized that anyone else had tried it until many years later when I had a coronary thrombosis. During my convalescence a woman priest used to bring me the sacraments and afterwards we had short discussions. I knew she was going through a difficult period and I mentioned these experiences to her. I was pleasantly surprised to learn that a parish priest had taught her a similar method of coping with the burden of other people's revelations.

Imipramine came into general use when I was at Whitchurch hospital. This was the first drug to be helpful in the treatment of clinical depression, and it seemed to me that the best place to use it was in general practice. Twelve months had passed since I had joined the hospital staff. I had recovered my inner composure and felt confident that I could make the grade of consultant psychiatrist if I so wished, but I now felt that I should return to general practice and in 1960 I was fortunate to be offered a post at Llanidloes, an ancient market town in a beautiful part of rural Wales. I later learnt that the senior partner was a great admirer of Sir Wilfred Grenfell.

Country Doctor

I have worked in many different medical posts, but the position that suited me best was that of a country doctor. I joined two older practitioners in Llanidloes, where we had our own cottage hospital and did most things, apart from major surgery, including attending all births and road traffic accidents. The nearest District Hospital was thirty miles away and in winter the road was sometimes closed by heavy snowfalls. *Dr Finlay's Casebook* was a popular television programme of that period. This fictional series portrayed the life of an elderly Scottish GP, Dr Cameron, and his young assistant Dr Finlay, and patients would sometimes remark on the similarity of their relationship and that between my senior partner and myself. This was not really surprising, but many people, including my partners, were surprised that I went to church regularly each Sunday. For me it was an essential part of my life and later my wife chose to accompany me together with our young children.

At Llanidloes I had many opportunities to develop my interest in spinal manipulation. We saw a lot of back problems: they usually resolved with bed rest and analgesics, but I now began to use some of the chiropractic techniques that Dr Cyriax had taught in his outpatient clinics at St Thomas's Hospital in the 1950s. Patients seemed to improve more quickly with manipulation and later I attended a short course on osteopathy at the Robert Jones and Agnes Hunt Hospital, Gobowen. I liked the gentleness of this approach and was confident enough to use it on patients when I felt it would help.

I also practised hypnotherapy. I had taught myself to hypnotize subjects many years previously, but had never bothered to develop this ability into a therapeutic tool until a midwife suggested that it might be helpful during childbirth. She volunteered to be my first hypnotherapy subject and the result was sufficiently encouraging for me to offer hypnotherapy as an aid to pain relief to the mothers who came to me for maternity care. Only one elected not to take advantage of the opportunity. She was a follower of the Maharishi and was concerned at the effect the procedure might have on her spiritual development. My main problem with hypnotherapy was that it required more time than I could allocate to it; consequently, I used it only as an adjuvant to other forms of analgesia.

The 1960s saw a burgeoning of hippie culture. Many 'flower people' were attracted to mid-Wales and the ones I met tended to have a gentle spirituality about them which I found attractive. Most lived in small communes and, if they were patients, I would sometimes visit them in their homes. I remember delivering a baby in an Ouspensky commune; it was an easy delivery watched by the mother's sister sitting cross-legged on the floor. I could not help noticing the lingering scent of cannabis in some houses but apart from choosing to have their babies delivered at home instead of hospital, their approach to medical care was conventional, with no obvious bias to alternative therapies. That came later.

The few patients who were opposed to conventional treatment were usually of farming stock. They would discuss their problems with me and when the various possibilities had been examined decide to just 'trust in the Lord'. In most instances there was no urgent need for treatment, but it was sad to learn that a woman I knew well had died from breast cancer many years later, having deliberately concealed the growth from her doctors and a daughter who was a nurse. Subsequently her daughter committed suicide.

The Church and Medicine

The inhabitants of Llanidloes are very tolerant of other people's beliefs. It was there that I first attended Eastern Orthodox services and Quaker meetings, and was privileged to be one of the first lay people to read a lesson in a Catholic church. This was soon after Vatican 2 and Fr Gillespie used me as a catalyst in his efforts to involve his parishioners more closely in the ritual of the mass. On another occasion I was asked to preach on St Luke's Day in the parish church. I wanted to decline but said 'yes' and found myself standing before a much larger congregation than usual. Shortly afterwards I was asked to take a service at the Baptist Chapel and various other requests followed to lead services in remote hillside chapels. I would always do so, but found that the commitment required a great deal of preparation and I realized that this was not an activity to which I felt particularly drawn. Shortly before leaving Llanidloes I was invited to preach at the parish church again. This was an ecumenical service and the subject of my address, as early as 1972, was 'Faith Healing'. I then predicted that the time would come when healing services would be held in that church; this expectation has since been validated.

My church attendance drew some interesting comments, particularly from children. One of the remarks I like best was told to me by the grandmother of a young boy whose mother had taken him to his first church service on Easter Sunday. On this occasion I was assisting the celebrant by offering the chalice to the communicants. His grandmother had stayed behind to cook the lunch and when they returned home she was full of questions, wanting to know whether he had enjoyed himself and what had happened. The boy was noncommittal then, after lunch, he suddenly said, 'I saw Dr Rees today. He was standing at the end of the church giving the people their medicine.' He could not have made a more penetrating comment, because that was the way I felt about it.

Another incident also involved a grandchild. I had visited an old lady at home and a few days later her son came to tell me what had happened after my visit. Apparently his young daughter had commented on the situation by saying, 'If Dr Rees cannot cure nain [gran], then we will have to ask Jesus to do it for us.' I can't say if Jesus' help was invoked, but the old lady did recover from her illness.

I was not particularly prayerful about my patients, but sometimes the situation evoked that response. I was called late at night to see an elderly lady in a residential nursing home. I was met by the matron who took me up a spiral staircase to the room she occupied. When we entered I saw that she was desperately ill. She was comatose, stertorous and very breathless. She was too ill to move and the best I could do was to give her some intravenous aminophylline, which only made her worse. She now became more deeply unconscious and began to vomit a large quantity of blackish fluid. We managed to turn her onto her side so that she did not inhale too much of the vomit and then waited to see what happened. During this time, as I sat on the bed, I offered a quiet inward prayer, not for her recovery but for her soul, then we left the room and I asked matron to phone me in the morning to let me know how she was. Next morning when matron phoned, I said that I would take the death certificate to her, but she said it was not necessary as the patient had recovered fully. When I next saw her she was standing at the top of the staircase smiling down at me. She was alive and well when I left Llanidloes. I never spoke to her about the incident.

There were some lovely people in the area. Mr and Miss Jarman were siblings who were still living in the farmhouse where they had been born over ninety years before. It was an isolated farm in a Welsh valley, without any modern facilities, not even a well — their water came from the mountainside through a pipe fixed in the bank some thirty yards from the house. They thought the water was wonderful and always encouraged me to drink it whenever I visited them. Drunk straight from the pipe it was always icy cold.

They had never needed any medical care and I was the first doctor to visit them since their early childhood when they were vaccinated against the 'coopox', their word for the smallpox vaccination. The Jarmans had always been members of the Church in Wales, not 'chapel people' like most Welsh farmers. They had a high regard for the role of the vicar, which they pronounced 'ficer', and Miss Jarman would sometimes say to me 'you should be a ficer', which she obviously considered a more important position than that of doctor. In her younger days, an old lady had given her a formula for an ointment that would cure most skin problems, and she passed it on to me. It must have been a very old prescription, dating back at least to the early nineteenth century. It contained three ingredients: equal parts of goose fat, lanolin and lard. Miss Jarman had found it helpful for a variety of skin complaints but I never used it so I cannot say how effective it might have been. Another farmer informed me that wormwood was a certain cure for jaundice. I was not tempted to follow his advice even when we had a localized epidemic among the children. They all recovered with no other treatment than the nursing care given by their mothers.

Research in General Practice

I am probably a workaholic. I am also intuitive and inquisitive. The combination of these attributes enabled me to undertake a surprising amount of research work even though the Llanidloes practice was extremely busy and we had very little free time. In some ways this was a pioneering enterprise as very few GPs were interested in research in the 1960s and there were no support networks or funding for such projects. All the costs of the research I paid for, but this did not seem to matter. Those now working in the various branches of healing who may be interested in research probably face similar problems to those that existed in general practice forty years ago. But the situation is changing rapidly and funding is increasingly becoming available to those who understand the system. Such people are most likely to be found working in academic departments of complementary medicine, nursing and general practice.

Between 1965 and 1972 I published ten original articles,[3-12] possibly more than any other GP in the UK at that time. Of these, seven appeared in the *British Medical Journal*. They covered a wide range of topics, including bereavement, depression, the effects of being struck by lightning during pregnancy, the distress of dying, the illnesses of motorists and the attendance of GPs at road traffic accidents. Two of the papers had some influence on subsequent developments. One dealt with tractor accidents. It appeared in the *British Medical Journal* in 1965 and showed that if a tractor overturned and the driver was injured the probability of his being killed was 1 in 4. It was the first publication to look closely at this problem and it advised that tractors should be provided with safety frames strong enough to protect the driver should the vehicle overturn. This was in contrast to the advice being given by government officials, who claimed that agricultural tractors were safe and that any mishaps were the fault of the drivers. Soon after the paper appeared, Parliament passed a law making the attachment of safety cabs a legal requirement on all new agricultural tractors produced in the UK, and I like to think that my paper helped to hasten the passing of that law. About eighty people were being killed each year by overturning tractors in 1965. I believe the figure now is closer to five.

Of more general interest was the paper on 'The Hallucinations of Widowhood', which the *British Medical Journal* published in 1971. This was a study I undertook with Sylvia Lutkins, a statistician at Aberystwyth University, but she kindly allowed the paper to be headed by my name only, as it was the subject of my MD thesis. This paper received a lot of publicity and its findings have been replicated in other centres. It dealt with the subjective experiences of the bereaved and showed that about 50 per cent of widowed people have a 'sense of the presence of their dead spouse' and that this is a normal and helpful consequence of widowhood. Psychiatrists accept the validity of these findings and people are much more likely to discuss them than previously, but some Christians, particularly in the evangelical churches, still tell people that these perfectly normal experiences are a form of demonic possession, which needs to be treated by 'deliverance'. This is a most perverse viewpoint and its implications will be discussed later in this book. But it is not only evangelical Christians who are convinced of the reality of demonic possession. The Catholic and Anglican Churches have exorcists to deal with evil spirits and more significantly the casting out of demons is widely practised as a healing technique in non-Christian cultures.

It was at Llanidloes that I learned to dowse, a skill valued by many homeopaths, though I do not practise this branch of medicine myself. Dowsing has given me a lot of fun though I rarely use the procedure now and could not be sure of locating underground water without a great deal of practice. I should also add that my interests in religion and medicine are eclectic, and I prefer to find areas of agreement in these disciplines rather than points of difference, whilst accepting that such differences exist and are important.

Back to England

In 1974 I left Llanidloes. Since then I have often been asked, 'Why did you go?' There were many reasons but my standard reply is to say, 'It was folly'. There is no doubt that I was overstretched and needed a long break. In addition to the practice work, I was much involved with the Church in Wales, being a member of various synods and of the Governing Body and was writing regular reports and 'position papers' on aspects of bereavement for people in the United States. I needed a holiday and when that situation arises I find it easier to change my job. At this crucial time, quite suddenly and unexpectedly, I was offered the post of senior lecturer at a London medical school. We visited the department and I decided not to accept the offer but it was unsettling, and when the possibility arose of joining a prestigious unit in London with a large multidisciplinary research project I was interested. Moreover, from the family and practice perspective, the timing seemed appropriate. The practice was scheduled to move into a new, purpose-built centre and would no longer require the surgery that was part of my house. My daughters were away at school and my son seemed quite eager to leave Llanidloes. My wife was in agreement and so I accepted the post of Senior Medical Officer in the Civil Service Department in central London.

The new post had various attractions, including civil service holidays, free weekends, no night duties, a splendid office and the opportunity to work on a large research project. The disadvantages included a long train journey into London from our base in Newbury and the sudden escalation of house prices. At Newbury I met Percy Corbett, a retired civil servant and member of the Church of England who was also secretary of the Churches' Fellowship for Psychical and Spiritual Studies. He knew a great deal about healing and spiritualism and with him I went to a Spiritualist church and met members of the National Federation of Spiritualist Healers, who allowed me to attend their healing clinics and practise healing with them. The atmosphere at these healing sessions was open, chatty and friendly, not secretive or bizarre in any way. I was apprehensive about attending a Spiritualist church, but Valerie and I went together and neither of us found anything disturbing about the proceedings.

In London, I also took the opportunity of visiting the Royal Homeopathic Hospital and was the first doctor to be allowed to attend teaching sessions at the nearby London School of Osteopathy. I only went a few times, but was impressed by the teaching given and the friendliness of the students. At the same time, I was encouraged by my employers to spend half a day each week with Dr Webb-Peploe, consultant cardiologist at St Thomas's Hospital, and learnt a great deal from him also. But I was becoming quite worried about our financial position. It was a time of rapid inflation, house prices were escalating and we no longer owned a property. Eventually, I realized that I must return to general practice and, against the wishes of my family, obtained a post as a single-handed GP in a Warwickshire village. I also became medical officer to Princethorpe College, a Catholic boarding school, and to the Police Training Centre at Ryton-on-Dunsmore.

Four years later I was offered the post of Medical Director at St Mary's Hospice in Birmingham and remained there for about ten years. I believe we practised holistic medicine at the hospice in its truest sense, providing care, to the best of our ability, for the patients' emotional, mental, physical, social and spiritual needs. This could not be done by individuals working alone; it was achieved by people of many disciplines working together. Most of the patients had cancer, but we were also involved in the care of patients with AIDS and motor-neurone disease and provided respite care for other very disabled people. Various forms of treatment were provided, including acupuncture, and some patients had attended the Bristol Cancer Centre, but the use of complementary medicine was not as extensive as it is today. The post involved a great deal of teaching, mainly in postgraduate medical centres and in hospitals, but we also ran our own English National Board courses for nurses and I was sometimes asked to talk to them about alternative therapies, which I did quite happily. I also had regular sessions with medical students from the University of Birmingham and the University recognized my contribution in this field by appointing me Honorary Senior Clinical Lecturer. Working in the hospice was extremely stressful and I was glad to be able to retire at the age of sixty, much earlier than I would have expected had I remained in general practice. Soon afterwards I had a coronary thrombosis and later required coronary angioplasty for unstable angina pectoris. I must thank Dr Martin Been and his team at the Walsgrave Hospital for the skilled and prompt care that enabled me to survive these critical moments.

Coventry Cathedral

When I was working in Birmingham, we continued to live in the Warwickshire village of Stretton-on-Dunsmore, which is close to the city of Coventry and its famous cathedral. Valerie and I belong to the cathedral community and one of my retirement activities is to act as a cathedral guide and share with people from all over the world the glories of that wonderful building and its message of forgiveness and reconciliation, which is so essential for the healing both of individuals and communities.

Being part of the cathedral community brought me into contact with the Very Revd John Petty the Provost, and subsequently first Dean, of Coventry Cathedral. John's enthusiasm for healing rekindled my interest in the subject and I appreciated anew the important function the Church has to bring healing to society. When Mr Alf Youell, with some other benefactors, financed the establishment of a healing centre, with its own chapel, kitchen and counselling rooms, at the cathedral I was gently drawn into this ministry. Then, to my surprise, I was asked to continue leading the services when John retired and have continued to do so for the past few years. In this work I do not set myself up as a healer but as a member of a group ministry.

Healing services can vary a great deal in style and content: ours are quiet, meditative occasions in which every one is involved in the laying on of hands and in receiving healing. Many of the people who attend these services have no other contact with the cathedral and whilst we cannot claim any spectacular miracles, people often say that they feel better for being there and, in some instances, it is obvious that they have improved quite dramatically.

Before John Petty retired, Coventry City Council suggested having a day conference on healing, for older people, in the cathedral. This was arranged and I became involved in the organization of the event, which was sold out in a few days of its being advertised. The conference included key note addresses by John Petty and Sarida Brown, editor of *Caduceus* and head of the Sufi healing order in the United Kingdom. There were demonstrations and talks by an aromatherapist, an acupuncturist, a member of the Brahma Kumaris, a Muslim and a Reiki master. This inclusive attitude to healing is central to this book. It is an approach that is second nature to most doctors who are constantly working with people from different ethnic backgrounds. We learn to welcome the inputs they provide and the different lessons they can teach us. Inevitably, the theological mind tends to be more exclusive. Here the emphasis is on working within the boundaries of faith and discerning the differences between creeds that enables devotees to feel certain of the correctness of their position compared with others. This leads inevitably to tension when matters of healing impinge on those of faith. For instance, this week I met an Asian lady whom I had helped a few years ago when she was going through a psychotic episode. We both attended a Eucharist and the next day a Christian healing service. She also goes to the Brahma Kumaris centre and the local university where she attends a course on stress management. She is seeking help from a range of agencies and I regard this as a sensible way of dealing with her problems. I am also aware that some religious people would find fault with her approach and the simultaneous acceptance of spiritual support from separate Hindu and Christian centres. I find this very sad. We do not have a monopoly of loving care in the West and it is far wiser to be open to the contribution that other cultures can make. I feel that there is much to learn from the ways different societies treat their sick. We shall consider some of these in the next chapter.

Chapter Two
Healing in Different Cultures

The concept of the healing priest is a reflection of the close association between the practice of religion and medicine and is found throughout recorded history. Societies have always cared for their sick to the best of their ability, and from very early times the 'healer' or 'shaman' or 'witch doctor' has had a very distinctive role within the tribe (or community), combining as he did the mystical elements of both traditions. The ultimate expression of this concept was made manifest in Christ, the archetypal healer and, according to the Letter to Hebrews, the eternal High Priest.

The earliest recorded physician-priest is Imhotep, Grand Vizier to the Egyptian Pharaoh some 5,000 years ago. In Europe, the first great healer was Hippocrates (c 460–370 BCE), a Greek physician, who belonged to a family of priests and doctors based on the island of Kos, where he practised his art and where the ruins of his temple still attract many visitors. His influence was so enduring that for many centuries he was called the father of medicine and the Hippocratic Oath remained the basis of medical conduct until quite recently.

Central to the Hippocratic code is the declaration that the doctor will do no harm to his patient or to an unborn foetus; that he will not abuse his privileged status; and will respect a patient's privacy. Perhaps the greatest difference between Hippocratic medicine and modern medicine is that the former focused solely on the relationship between the doctor and his patient, but nowadays the wider concerns of society are also taken into consideration. Hippocrates advised people to eat and drink in moderation, to let nature take its course and to live where the air is good. He also stressed the need for cleanliness in both physicians and patients.

Like many modern healers, Hippocrates believed that a healing energy – he called it the *vix medicatrix naturae* – circulated in the body and that disease occurred if the internal balance of the body was disrupted. Like the modern psychiatrist, he was also interested in people's personalities and taught that there were four basic personality types – the sanguine, the choleric, the

17

phlegmatic and the melancholic – which were related to one of the four elements – earth, air, fire and water – which were believed at the time to form
the universe. There were also four bodily 'humours' – blood, phlegm, black
bile and yellow bile – and he believed that health depended on keeping these
humours in balance, a concept that is very similar to that of practitioners of
Ayurvedic medicine, though they speak of *doshas*, not humours.

Some of the distinctive features of Ayurvedic medicine and of traditional Chinese medicine will be discussed later, but it is important to point out
here that these ancient forms of medical care remain an essential part of
the health care systems in Asia, even though modern Western medicine is
also widely available. Most Ayurvedic practitioners work in the rural areas
of India and provide health care for at least 500 million people in that
country alone. The Indian Medical Council recognizes the important role
they play in providing public welfare and, since 1971, has conferred academic qualifications on graduates in Ayurvedic medicine: it also
appreciates the contribution of other forms of traditional medical practice
in India such as Unani and Siddha.

The Chinese also have a high regard for their system of traditional medicine, and this is a particularly important resource for those living in rural areas.
All medical schools are encouraged to form links with colleges of Chinese medicine and to teach traditional medicine as part of their curriculum.

African Countries

Africa is a vast continent with many nations, tribes and different cultures.
Economically, it is a very deprived area and most African governments have
little money to spare for public health projects. A disproportionately high per-
centage of the world's sick live in these poor countries and, of these, a high
proportion are children. There is much malnutrition and anaemia, and many
deaths from diseases which have been almost eliminated in more affluent
societies. HIV/AIDS is rife and, according to a United Nations prediction,
half of all teenagers in some African countries will die of AIDS at an early age.[1]

In many parts of Africa, 80–90 per cent of the population consult traditional healers; in South Africa over 75 per cent do so. Traditional healers
are often the only source of health care and some governments are using
this fact in a positive manner. The Tanzanian University of the Health
Sciences offers a course in traditional medicine, and government-sponsored courses for traditional healers are helping to improve the
effectiveness of the AIDS prevention programmes in Mozambique and
Zambia. In South Africa, the possibility of integrating Western and traditional medicine is being discussed and the Department of Health is also
seeking to establish a Traditional Healer Council.[2]

All traditional African cultures have a magico-spiritual concept of disease. This does not allow for the possibility that death may be the result of purely natural causes: it is always believed to have been brought about by another agency, usually human, and most commonly by means of magic or witchcraft. Mbiti explains it in this way:

> if a child dies from malaria, the mother will not be satisfied with the explanation that a mosquito, carrying malarial parasites, stung the child and caused it to die. She will wish to know why the mosquito stung her child and not somebody else's. The only satisfactory answer is that 'someone' sent the mosquito or worked some other evil magic against her child. This is not a scientific answer but it is a reality for the majority of African people.[3]

As a consequence, attempts will be made, probably with the help of a witchdoctor, to identify the person responsible so that they can be confronted and made to make reparation.

Traditional healers have a multifaceted role. They act as herbalist, psychologist, priest, ceremonial leader, seer and physician in one. They understand and share the belief systems of their people. This includes the certainty that the spiritual world intertwines closely with this earthly world. For Africans, spirits are a reality that must be reckoned with: there are nature spirits, which inhabit trees, fields, hills, mountains and stretches of water; there are also demi-gods and spirits whose special concern is with the nation or tribe itself. The most important spirits though are those of the 'living dead', the recently deceased ancestors. The community and individual members themselves have to perform various rites to maintain a good relationship with these spirit entities, including the sacrifice of animals, offerings of food or the pouring of libations of beer, milk, water or coffee. They believe that if they fail in this duty, the individual, family or tribe may suffer. Such beliefs are unacceptable to many Western people, but they are not so widely different from the Christian concept of the 'communion of saints' or the 'great cloud of witnesses', mentioned in the Letter to Hebrews.

Dancing and clapping are part of the healing ritual in most African cultures. The Bushmen believe these activities release an energy, *Num*, which travels up the spine to the top of the head and enables individuals – most notably the witchdoctor – to become 'possessed' and travel to the spirit world where they can discuss the patient's health with the ancestors. While 'possessed', the witch doctor may gyrate, scream, shake uncontrollably and fall down. When he regains normal consciousness, he is likely to seize the individual so as to extract the infirmity and cast it away. This is painful and exhausting work and is supported by the community in its dance. It is the dance that activates the *Num* that heals the afflicted.

The Yaka of Zaire

The Yaka are a small tribe of casual labourers, hunters and subsistence farmers who live in West Africa. They believe that healing is largely a matter of self-healing, and that this can be achieved by the performance of appropriate rituals. They do not perceive illness in the way that Europeans do, as being due to infections or cancerous tumours or disturbances of the immune system, they regard it as a loss of *m-mooyi*, one's vital energy. This force is seen as an élan vital which distinguishes the individual from everyone else yet links them with the rest of the tribe: it is an asexual essence of personal, social and cosmological significance. Illness occurs when a fault in the individual's relationships with other members of the tribe, or with the spirits, causes the *m-mooyi* to leak away. Healing is 'making whole the loss, and re-establishing the damaged social and cosmological interfaces'.[4] There are echoes here of Archbishop William Temple's dictum that 'The Kingdom of Heaven is the sum of right relationships'.

Healing rituals are community events. They tend to be highly dramatic occasions in which everyone in the village, 100–200 people, is involved. The *khita*, or gynaecological ritual, is one such example. The focal point of the action is the *fula*, a wooden stick, which symbolizes both the patient's problem and the sap of the palm tree. The main participants in the ceremony are the patient, her husband, an uncle and the therapist. They enact a struggle over the *fula*, the symbol of male virility. Attached to the stick are small bags containing items which may have been stolen and cursed, and which are believed to have brought about her present condition. All four participants grasp the *fula*, thumping it rhythmically against the ground, chanting a series of woes that need to be rectified, and outlining the patient's past and present problems. Towards the end of the struggle the woman becomes entranced and, having won possession of the stick, is encouraged to recount her grievances and the circumstances associated with her illness more fully.

The ritual is cathartic, enabling the patient to unleash all her pent-up emotions whilst at the same time infusing new meaning into her situation. The stick, which started as the symbol of male virility, now becomes a sign of liberated fertility and fertilization. By hugging the stick closely, she links her 'dying' in the trance to her former illness, and her 'rebirth' into clear consciousness, to her recovery. The ritual also provides her with a greater degree of bisexuality and with it an increased capacity for self-realization. Although the other three participants are male, during the ceremony they also show signs of social bisexuality, so the healing ritual combines both male and female elements.[5]

Witchdoctors in the Philippines

Most Third World healers have an animistic philosophy. This is certainly evident in the Philippines where they invoke discarnate spirits in their fight against disease. In its book *Health, Healing and Wholeness*, the Salvation Army looks with great candour at this aspect of life in that country. It points out that whilst Filipino Salvationists have given up alcohol, drugs, smoking and other social vices: 'It is not uncommon to see some Salvationists, including officers, submitting to diviners in their quest for health and healing. They believe that their daily life is most often influenced by spirits, whether the Holy Spirit or evil spirits.' When sick, in common with other Filipino Christians, Salvationists ask three questions.

1. What is the physical cause of the sickness?
2. What have I done to get this sickness?
3. Who did this to me?

If they decide that the complaint is purely physical, they will go to a 'doctor', usually a 'folk practitioner', who will prescribe herbal medicines and a powerful prayer that the patient has to recite. When the sick feel that they themselves are to blame, they will pray to God for forgiveness and promise to do better and make amends. If both these options are rejected, they will assume that an enemy has paid a spirit doctor to make them ill. They will then set about employing their own witch doctor to remove the curse. The healing ritual will include the sacrifice of an animal whose blood is used to paint crosses on and around the house as a protection against the evil spirits, all done to the accompaniment of dancing and the chanting of prayers. Finally, the animal is either burnt as an offering to the spirits or buried under the house.[6]

Healing in Puerto Rico

In Puerto Rico, spiritualistic healing offers an acceptable and traditional alternative to other modes of health care. Almost everyone in the country has had some contact with spiritualism and about 60 per cent of people, of all socioeconomic groups, visit a *centro* (spiritualist centre) at some time. Many health professionals – doctors, nurses, psychologists and social workers – come from families of spirit healers (mediums) and some manage to work in both fields simultaneously, combining the role of a modern therapist (a nurse, for example) with that of a traditional healer.[7]

In Puerto Rico the healers are mainly older women of the same social class as the patient. They are considered to have special attributes, including great empathy with the sick and extensive knowledge of the spirits. Their role as healers is validated by significant, often ecstatic, experiences and consequently they are regarded as vehicles of divine authority and so are much more powerful than their patients. Their healing expertise is derived from a quasi-religio-philosophical system, called *Espiritisimo*, which originated in France and is based on the teachings of Leon Rivail (1803–69), a scholar and writer whose ideas reached Latin America mainly through Spain.

Healing usually takes place in public, in a group setting, which anyone can attend free of charge. The healers receive spirit messages or become possessed by the spirits before they diagnose, counsel, prescribe and prognosticate. Many people attend the sessions, but only a few are selected from the audience for healing. The healer first observes the patient, and then describes what is wrong. She assimilates the problem into her own body and, if she divines the illness as being 'physical' rather than 'spiritual', she will refer the patient to a medical doctor, though she will expect the patient to return to her after consulting the physician so that she can retain overall control. There is a certain overlapping of responsibility anyway, as many patients consult both doctors and healers at the same time, sometimes for complex reasons, such as their need to have a social explanation for a medically treatable disease.

The *centro* caters mainly for people with family problems, nervous complaints, headaches, backaches, bad dreams or stress-related disorders. The healer almost invariably includes the patient's family in the diagnosis and treatment of these conditions. Helpful advice is likely to be given in a cosmological and life-affirming context. Healers often insist on patients developing new coping strategies and then pursuing personal transformation, possibly with the view to their becoming healers themselves. Specific treatments may include the performance of exorcistic rites, which are conducted by the healer, and the prescription of herbal remedies. The healer will also encourage the patient to adopt a more prayerful attitude to life.

The Incas

The Philippines and Puerto Rico were colonized by Spain in the sixteenth century but survive as independent states with their own distinctive cultures. Other societies have disappeared so completely that our knowledge of their customs and beliefs is very sparse. Such is the case with the Inca empire, which dominated south-west America until it was overthrown by Pizarro in 1533. Physical evidence of their civilization includes the ruins of palaces and temples, statues and sculptured decorations. The Incas built good roads, had a well-developed system of agriculture and were skilled in

the making of ceramics and textiles. They were an intelligent and sophisticated people who worshipped the sun and, not surprisingly, their
understanding of illness and healing was quite different from ours. It is
best understood in relation to their cosmology – their perception of the
nature of society and the role of the individual within it, most importantly
the relationship of humanity and the sanctified forces of nature with the
supernatural spheres. In this, their beliefs were very close to those of the
Yaka of West Africa.

Central to Incan philosophy was the concept of *ayni*, a term embracing
both balance and reciprocity. Health, both social and individual, was
regarded as being intrinsically linked with the maintenance of a balance
between natural and supernatural forces. Disease was the result of a breakdown of this unifying equilibrium, and individuals by their wrong-doing
could not only harm themselves and society, but also instigate natural dis-
asters like floods and earthquakes.

The traditional healers of Incan society functioned as both herbalists
and priests. They were extremely knowledgeable about the medicinal properties of plants, they practised divination and acted as confessors, and they
also directed the ritual cleansing which supplicants required before they
were fit to make offerings to the ancestors and the gods. Some healers specialized in treating patients with herbs, others as bonesetters or
soothsayers, the latter often chewing tobacco or coca before making their
predictions. One of the healing rites was called 'feeding' the deities. The
sick would be given ground corn and seashells, on which they would blow
so as to offer them as a gift to the gods, asking for health as they did so. In
the same way, coca would be blown to the sun,[8] moon and stars to obtain
harmony and health.

The Conjurors of Wales

Every country has its own tradition of folk medicine. In some it remains
vibrant and active, in others it has almost completely disappeared and
remains only as a folk memory. In my own country of Wales the traditional healers were the Physicians of Myddfai and the conjurors. The former
were medieval doctors of outstanding ability, whilst the conjurors, inheri-
tors of a more recent tradition, continued to practise into the early
twentieth century. One famous conjuror was still operating in the 1940s.
He was Morris of the Vulcan Arms, Cwmbelan, a hamlet in an area where
I worked as a general practitioner in the 1960s and where the older patients
would occasionally speak of him.

There was probably no real conflict of interest between the local medical practitioners and the conjurors. The former were consulted mainly for

'matters of life and death', the latter for the daily problems of people including the care of their sick kinsfolk and animals. To be successful, they had to have a shrewd understanding of local affairs and of the men and women who came to them for help. Robert Gibbins, an Irish academic, said this of the conjurors of Mid-Wales in 1943:

> But the real point is that the conjuror was wise. And there are conjurors alive today who can work miracles when all the powers of science fail. Indeed, it is whispered that members of the university agricultural departments have visited these men on dark nights to seek cures for troubles that have baffled them. And with success.[9]

Gibbins knew Morris and visited him at the Vulcan Arms, where he worked as a blacksmith. He kept a hut by the smithy for those waiting for their horses and, as it was a farming area, the conversation would be about sheep, tractors and politics, but Morris was just as knowledgeable about poetry, astronomy and natural history.

An elderly lady told me of his visits to her parents' farm when she was a child. She recalled her mother taking him into the sitting room – not the kitchen where people usually went – and leaving him there alone. Being an inquisitive child she crept to the closed door, peeped through the keyhole and saw him sitting at the table, writing. Her mother scolded her for this, but she remembers that when Morris left the house he handed over the paper and her mother pushed it into a hole in an enclosure wall. Many years later the wall collapsed and in one section they found a bottle which contained the prescriptions that Morris had written. These were in the form of an alchemical charm and it was the custom to place them near the site of the trouble: in a boundary wall for worries about the sheep, in the barn for cattle, and in the rafters of the house for family problems.

Morris had a book which he consulted when healing. After his death it was deposited in the manuscript department of the National Library of Wales, Aberystwyth, where it can be read. It is entitled *The Art of Talismanic Magic. Being Selections from the Works of Rabbi Solomon, Agrippa, Barrett etc.* and is dated 1888. A simple exercise book with lined paper, it contains handwritten extracts from what is probably a sixteenth-century hermeneutic treatise. It starts by telling the aspirant how he should live and that:

- He must apply himself with the utmost attention to this art.
- Be sober and detached from the pleasures of a debauched life. Be learned in astrology.
- Be firm and steadfast.
- Have some discreet Person who will encourage and animate you. Be confident and certain of success.

It also stipulates the proper places and times for studying. These include:

- A retired place remote from the hurry of business. Silent and tranquil solitude.
- A small room to which none has access. It should be simply furnished and the furniture should be new and sprinkled with holy water. It should be kept with the greatest decency and cleanliness.
- The best time is 'the rising of the sun'.

A 'knowledge of astrology' was a normal requirement for physicians in the Middle Ages, but there is also an interesting emphasis on the need for sobriety, quietness and both ritual and physical cleanliness. Much of the book is concerned with the use and making of talismans, which could be fashioned in metal or parchment. The book ends with the admonition:

> Who ever attempts to understand the Great Mysteries Let him live up to the teachings of Christ Jesus. His Redeemer and Saviour. Who died for the sins of all.[10]

This affirmation of Christian belief was written by someone who appears to have been involved in magical practices, but we have to bear in mind that such a syncretism was probably commonplace in the Middle Ages, when physicians were expected to be skilled in the art of astrology and other practices that might be considered inappropriate for medical practitioners today.

George Lloyd was another healer who lived in the locality. Robert Gibbins consulted him with chronic backache, a problem that had troubled him for over a year. They met in the back kitchen of a farmhouse, a room hung with saddles, spurs and sheep shears, and for the first quarter of an hour they just chatted about anything except the pain. Lloyd, a middle-aged man with quiet grey eyes, eventually asked Gibbins for his full name. Then he took a ball of wool, tied a knot in the end and, placing the knot on his elbow, measured three lengths with his finger and thumb. He did this three times. He then broke the thread, folded it up, wrapped it in brown paper, gave it to Gibbins and told him to tie it on his left leg next to the skin and leave it there until it fell off. Then he should burn it. Lloyd also told him that the pain would be gone within a week. The next morning Gibbins felt much better, the pain disappeared within a week and did not return.[11]

Anthropologists and Healers

Our understanding of the role of healers in traditional societies has been greatly enhanced by the work of social anthropologists. Their studies are becoming increasingly significant as former practices disappear, together with the local languages, dialects and oral traditions that enriched many cultures. Just as psychologists divide people into extroverts and introverts, so anthropologists classify traditional healers as being 'convergent or divergent', depending on the relationship they have with their patients and their status in the community. In the examples given, George Lloyd saw patients in the kitchen and had a relaxed friendly attitude: he was a 'convergent' healer. James Morris's approach was more distant and he was shown greater respect – he was taken into the sitting room – and should be classified as a 'divergent' healer. It so happens that both were men, but in many societies the healers are commonly, sometimes exclusively, women.

Convergent healers are ordinary people who are not easily distinguished from the rest of society. They do the same sort of work, speak in the same patois or dialect and dress in a similar fashion. They receive little or no formal training, but have developed their own innate abilities and have acquired their specialized knowledge by listening to reminiscences about the old ways, and by observing people and nature. Women are often not recognized as healers until they reach the menopause, for it is only then that they are regarded as being ritually clean and fit, therefore, for the role of archetypal mother, capable of mediating with the intangible worlds.

Divergent healers are usually set apart from the rest of the community. The most obvious modern counterpart is the hospital doctor or nurse, but in primitive societies they were the shamans or witchdoctors, who also acted as intermediaries between the living and the dead. This was not a role that they chose but one to which they felt they had been called, as still happens in many parts of the world today. The call to a special vocation would come in a vision, a dream or during a spiritual ecstasy, and there was often a preceding illness that helped to make the individual empathetic to those in need or who were ill. Shamans were most often men and while they prepared for their vocation would move away from the community and perhaps submit themselves to an arduous training regime. During this period they would change the way they dressed and behaved, and their speech would often acquire an accent and vocabulary different from that of the rest of the community. This tendency to acquire a particular profile is as apparent in divergent healers today as in the past.

Bajalica in the Balkans

The traditional healer in Serbia is called a *bajalica*, one who heals with words. They are 'convergent' healers, the gap between their social standing and that of their patients is small, and the healers are not obviously different from the rest of the community except in one important detail: *bajalicas* are invariably women and usually post-menopausal. Old women are ritually 'clean' and therefore safe and suitable recipients of the secret knowledge that is essential for the art. Their first task when consulted by a patient is to gain his/her trust, and this is done by talking with them and by establishing a close physical contact.

Erysipelas is a common problem in some rural communities and its management will serve as a good example of the way a *bajalica* and her patient interrelate. It is an infection of the skin caused by the haemolytic streptococcus and most often affects the face and lower legs. The patient suddenly feels ill and feverish, and develops a bright red, tender swelling, with a well-defined edge. The condition is self-limiting and will resolve by itself, but sometimes the infection becomes widespread and suppurates. If consulted, a doctor will prescribe penicillin but, in the countryside, sufferers often prefer to visit the *bajalica* for this complaint, which they call *crveni vetar*, the red wind. In Serbian folklore illnesses are caused by disease-bearing winds and the deep red inflammation of erysipelas is blamed on the red wind which has its origin 'out there', in the unknown regions which the *bajalica* understands.

At their first meeting the *bajalica* and her patient spend a great deal of time getting to know one another, and even if the patient is an older man he will address her as 'mother'. The healing ritual takes place over three days, usually in the kitchen or the farmyard, depending on the weather. The *bajalica* and patient always sit close together and any members of the family who may be present try to be unobtrusive. The meeting follows a definite pattern in an atmosphere that is relaxed and apparently unstructured. The *bajalica* is a skilled, almost hypnotic talker and her use of words and varied tones and inflections enables the patient to reach a state of altered consciousness where the 'red wind' is dispatched to the spirit world, the pain alleviated and a state of calmness attained.

Whilst the *bajalica* talks, she touches. Physical contact is an important aspect of Serbian culture and people will frequently touch one another whilst sitting or standing together. The curative touch is more subtle and gentle than normal physical contact. There is no haste; the healer takes her time and touches with her eyes before using the hands. Her hands are peasant hands, rough and work-worn, but she is careful to soften them with emollients when treating the sick. Physical closeness is part of the ritual and the healer will caress her patient with her voice, her breath and even her spittle.

Each part of the ritual is sealed by 'purification with fire'. The healer picks up a glowing ember from the fire and waves it in front of the patient. As the *bajalica* holds the ember in the space between them, they weave

their bodies in a sort of silent seated dance, which is both spontaneous and
all-knowing. Then the *bajalica* examines the wound, washes her hands with
rakija (homemade plum brandy) and with it cleans the wound, massaging
the inflamed area gently towards the heart which facilitates lymphatic
drainage. On the second day she rubs an ointment made of herbs, beeswax
and incense on the infected area, which is then wrapped in cloths. During
the three days of treatment the erysipelas visibly subsides. The infection
has been controlled, healing has been assured and the *bajalica*'s reputation
maintained. She recognizes that she draws her strength and authority from
a higher power and will say modestly '*Prvo bog pa ia*' ('First God then I').[12]

Ayurvedic Medicine

Many of the principles taught by the Hippocratic School are also to be
found in Ayurvedic medicine. This traditional system of health care has
been part of Indian culture for over 3,000 years and is widely practised in
other parts of Asia. Its basic concepts are probably derived from the *Vedas*,
the most sacred Hindu scriptures, and include the belief that everything in
the universe is composed of five elements – earth, air, fire, water and space
– which are collectively known as panchamahabhutas. The individual is
seen as being animated by three vital energies, or *doshas*, called *vatta*, *pitta*
and *kapha*. Whichever *dosha* predominates determines our *prakti*, or basic
personality, which is fixed at birth, but the stresses of life can distort the
balanced *prakti* into an imbalanced *vikrti*, and this can lead eventually to ill-
health. Like other healing systems, the aim of Ayurvedic medicine is to
prevent disease as well as cure it, and it stresses the need for a strict code
of personal and social hygiene. Preventive measures include following precise dietary rules and practising yoga. The treatments include diet,
purgation, bloodletting, the use of herbal medicines, head and body massage, and the application of ointments and liniments to the skin.

Some Ayurvedic practitioners work in Ayurvedic hospitals and it is now
possible to attend the Ayurvedic Charitable Hospital in London. Here a
course of treatment is likely to start with a full body massage using oils,
which may be followed by a herbal sauna when patients sit in a vertical bath
with their head sticking out of the lid. The facilities are good and yoga
classes and a variety of enemas are readily available.[13] One of the principles
of Ayurvedic medicine that practitioners like to emphasize is that the treatment must be tailored to the requirements of the patient.

Practitioners of Ayurvedic medicine are called *Vaids* and they are
responsible, in rural India, for the care of mentally disturbed patients as
well as those with physical complaints. They work on the principle that in
addition to the three humours – *vatta*, *pitta* and *kapha* – each person

possesses three psychic factors – *satwa* (light), *rajas* (activity) and *tamasa* (darkness) – and that a disturbance of the balance of these factors can lead to a psychiatric disorder. They also believe that over-activity of any of the humours, sexual overindulgence or the eating of unwholesome foods can also affect the mental equilibrium. *Vaids* classify foods as either 'cold' or 'hot'. Cold foods cause depression while hot ones tend to make people overexcited. They treat mental illness with Ayurvedic medicines, dietary advice and instructions about continence, but not usually with yoga. Sometimes they blame mental illness and fits on possession by evil spirits.

Practitioners of other styles of medicine also provide health care in rural India. Kapur found four categories of professional healers in a town of 10,000 people located between Bombay and Cape Cormoran. They were *vaids, mantarwadis, patris* and doctors practising Western medicine. This town supported twenty-six practitioners and of these two were *vaids*, three doctors, three *mantarwadis* and four *patris*; there were also fourteen other practitioners who called themselves *patrimantriks*, claiming to be both *mantarwadis* and *patris*. Four practitioners – one *vaid*, one doctor and two *mantarwadis* – had flourishing practices, the rest did less well.

The term healer does not describe the role of the *mantarwadis* and *patris* adequately. They certainly care for the sick, but people also consult them about business prospects, family relationships, the propitiation of rain gods and recovery of lost cattle. They base their work on Karmic principles, relating present misfortunes and illnesses to past actions, which the individual may have committed in this present life or in some previous incarnation. The unhappy consequences attributed to these misdeeds are sometimes explained in astrological terms – as a malign conjunction of the stars – or in demonic terminology – due to the intervention of spirits (*bhutas*) controlled by the god Shiva. Some *bhutas* are extremely malevolent causing disease and death, or they may take over a person's body, revealing their presence by epileptic fits or maniacal behaviour. Other *bhutas* are more playful, causing less serious disturbances.

Mantarwadis are astrologers who divine the basic problem with the help of a zodiacal chart. The consultation does not take place in private but in front of other clients, and the discussion is more likely to be focused on the cause of the problem than on its nature. The most frequently mentioned agent for any current misfortune is 'the displeasure of ancestral spirits', but blame is often attributed to the 'spirit of a dead child', to unfavourable alignments of the stars, to specific *bhutas* (all named) or to physical causes. The treatment provided by a *mantarwadi* is likely to be simple: the provision of a coloured thread to place around the wrist, some ash or a talisman. Patients may also be advised to visit a *bhuta* shrine as a penance.

A *patri* is a medium, and the spirit or demon who controls him conducts the therapeutic process. To the beating of drums and in an atmosphere rich with incense and the fragrance of areca flowers, the *patri* goes into a trance and is possessed by his master demon, who then confronts the client's demon. The client also goes into a trance and the two demons argue with one another and struggle for supremacy. If the *patri*'s demon wins, the client's demon is ordered to leave and does so. Should the client's demon be stronger, he is asked to state his conditions for leaving. These may be the holding of a ritual feast, an animal sacrifice or something similar.

Indian villagers will 'shop around' when they need treatment and, as in Western countries, they are likely to consult more than one healer. Women are more likely than men to consult Western-trained doctors and less likely to seek help solely from a traditional healer. It is worth noting that most people with psychiatric symptoms consult someone, a healer or a doctor, and this is particularly true if the symptoms are those of a psychosis or epilepsy, probably because of family pressure. Western-trained doctors work mainly in cities and are not readily accessible to villagers, but the latter prefer to consult a Western-trained doctor if possible. At the same time, the educated, the young and rich consult traditional healers just as often as the illiterate, the old and the poor.[14]

Healers in Indonesia

Indonesia has a population of 180 million people scattered over 3,000 islands. It has a well-developed health service, but traditional healers continue to play a key role in the provision of health care. There are 300 ethnic groups within the islands and many belief systems have influenced the development of traditional healing in the country. These include those of the original Malaysian culture, the now dominant Muslim religion, certain Chinese traditions, Buddhism, Hinduism, Christianity and even aspects of modern Western medicine. Some traditional healers like to carry stethoscopes, but the relationship between unconventional and orthodox medicine is a symbiotic one as some Western-style nurses and physicians also like to adopt a traditional therapeutic approach.

A useful pen portrait of indigenous healers is available in a government-sponsored review by Salan and Maretzki.[15] They looked at nine healers, three from each of the following localities: a Muslim region, a Hindu enclave in a Balinese region, and a Javanese centre with predominantly Muslim and Chinese healers. The healers all showed 'convergent' characteristics. Almost all the patients were from the lower or lower middle classes, and had the same schooling, religious affiliation and ethnicity as the healers. The latter often became healers after a severe illness, or following the death of a spouse or child, which had led to their becoming estranged from the rest of the community for a time. Some had a clear vocation having heard voices telling them to do so, but whatever the reason they invariably regarded healing as their primary activity and means of livelihood. As healers, they also invariably adopted whatever their former background, a parental attitude to their patients.

Indonesian healers place very few restrictions on their clients and usually allow patients to visit them at any time of the day or night. This is good business practice in a competitive field, but they also realize that the sick person may have walked many miles for the consultation. They always listen very carefully to what the patient says before attempting to diagnose and treat the complaint. They do this in various ways, but many practise trance possession. After going into a trance, healers may place a magnet or dagger over the body as an aid to diagnosis and then discuss the problem with the spirits. Non-trance healers will also use a dagger in this way, or they sometimes place metallic objects between the patient's fingers and touch them on the face, hands and painful spots, or place pieces of paper inscribed with quotations from the Holy Qur'ān on the body. When healers believe that the patient is afflicted by evil spirits they will recommend an exorcism; this is likely to include a ritual bath which the healer will perform at his home or at some sacred site, such as a holy cemetery. Some healers provide herbal medicines as part of the treatment, and may allow the patients to remain in their compounds for a few days while they are being treated. The exorcising ceremonies and some of the other traditional rituals can be very expensive but few Indonesian healers seem to gain much material benefit from their activities and, for many, payment for their services is not a particularly relevant issue. Others have a different attitude and demand a higher fee for the treatment provided than would most physicians.

Many healers will visit the patient's home to observe the family dynamics, but the initial consultation is always at the healer's house. Subsequent treatments may be given elsewhere, often at a site of symbolic significance such as a sacred place, which may enhance the therapeutic effect of the healing ritual. Patients rarely visit a healer alone; usually they are accompanied by members of the family or close friends. About half the patients who visit healers in Indonesia have self-limiting illnesses. The remainder suffer from chronic diseases, which may have troubled them for many years. A high proportion have psychological or psychiatric problems, including major mental disturbances. That said, 60 per cent of patients believe that their condition has improved following treatment,[16] and trance healers tend to have a higher success rate than non-trance healers. Healing linked to culturally based beliefs, with direct advice from supernatural beings, tends to be more effective than common-sense advice from non-trance healers.

Healers tend to show more care for their patients than hospital workers do. They listen more carefully to the patient and help by putting the illness into perspective. Many patients are really seeking advice, and healers give this in simple terms, and place it within the cultural ambience in which the patient feels most at ease. They reaffirm a traditional world-view that is meaningful to the patients, and do this not only with their explanations but also by the rituals they perform.[17] They also have sufficient knowledge of herbal remedies to suggest these when appropriate. A similar therapeutic approach was once typical of family doctors and community nurses in the UK, but this is no longer the case. Patients no longer have easy access to a medical consultation and with the increasing regimentation of the health service it is becoming easier for patients to make an appointment to see a complementary therapist than their own GP or practice nurse.

The *Zār Bori* of Northern Sudan

Indonesia is a mainly Muslim country and so is Sudan, but it is only in Sudan that the healing cult led by women for women, called the *Zār bori*, is to be found. It flourishes in an ethnically mixed area of northern Sudan dominated by the riverain group, a Muslim patriarchical society in which all decisions are made by men, all social functions are sharply defined and there is no sexual equality. Men control the finances, women care for the children and supervise the domestic sphere.[18] The riverain people place great emphasis on female virginity before marriage, and this is ensured by sexual segregation, close chaperonage and female 'circumcision' with infibulation. In extreme cases the infibulation is reinstated after childbirth so that a woman can return to her husband as if she were a virgin. The older women support these customs and supervise the operations.

A riverain girl can automatically expect to be the centre of attention and feted three times during her life: when she is infibulated, at her marriage and when she has children. If, however, she can obtain a *zār* healing she will again find herself the focus of elaborate ceremonies. Women are firmly in control of the *zār* ritual and the ceremonies associated with them, but they are very expensive and it is the husband who has to provide the necessary finance.

The people of northern Sudan suffer from many illnesses including a psychosomatic disease called *waham*, which occurs mainly in women. It is a common complaint, which usually presents as anxiety, depression, panic attacks or demonic possession. Fortunately, it is particularly amenable to ritual healing. When a woman's illness does not respond to the normal household remedies, she can seek help from three agencies. These are:

1. A member of the medical profession, usually a man.
2. A feki, or Qur'ānic healer, always male. He will use verses of the Qur'ān in different ways to treat the illness.
3. A leader of the zār cult – a woman.

The role of zār healer is one of the few occupations open to women in the Sudan, and leading healers tend to come from the lower strata of society and are often of slave descent. They are powerful individuals with good organizational ability, spiritual strength and considerable status among their peers. Their healing power is generally attributed to the special relationship they have with the spirits. Apart from their generally low social status, they also have a low sexual status, which some deliberately cultivate, often engineering their own divorce and refusing to be obedient and attractive to their husbands. They take the view that, because they are powerful healers and mediators with the spirits, they do not need husbands: and in order to remain close to the spirits, they should have nothing to do with such a degrading activity as sexual intercourse. Their low status gives them greater freedom as it enables them to visit freely and to receive into their houses strangers, including men, for the healing rituals.

A zār healing ceremony will last from one to seven days. The principal rite is centred on the patient and involves the burning of much incense, dressing up in costumes, dancing, drumming and singing. It is a deeply moving psychodrama in which the patient falls into a trance and becomes possessed by the spirits, as do others present at the ceremonies. All this has a pronounced cathartic effect and culminates in the sacrifice of a ram or billy-goat, a sacrifice which is quite explicitly a scapegoat for the patient. After the animal has been slaughtered the blood is used in the concluding rituals.

When the zār healing ritual is completed, the patient goes through the same elaborate cleansing rites that are mandatory after sexual intercourse, menstruation and childbirth. For some days she enters a state of semi-seclusion and is not required to perform any of her normal domestic duties. Then, before re-entering society, she bathes, cleans the skin again with perfumed smoke, and applies a scented paste called *dilka*. Finally, she dresses in fresh clothes, plaits her hair and resumes her normal role in the household. The *zār bori* is expensive and a wife has to be careful not to demand too many of these treatments from her husband but they are very effective.[19]

Male Circumcision

Although male circumcision cannot be described as a healing procedure it is certainly an excellent example of preventive medicine in action. The practice has a very long history and is an essential rite for Jewish and Muslim males. Its early association with Jewish beliefs is recorded in Genesis,[20] where the Creator God makes a covenant with Abraham requiring him to circumcise all male children, including slaves, when they are eight days old. The ancient Egyptians also circumcised boys, usually between the ages of six and twelve, and in many modern societies it is still performed ritually before puberty. Some groups even continue to use a stone knife in preference to a metal one, underlining further the antiquity of the operation.

In most instances circumcision is seen as a 'rite of passage', but in ancient civilizations the priests who performed this operation were also the doctors and it is likely that there were health implications even then. The practice offers protection against phimosis (restriction of the foreskin) and balanitis (inflammation of the foreskin). Recent studies show that circumcised men also have a lower incidence of sexually transmitted diseases – syphilis, gonorrhoea and HIV/AIDS – than the uncircumcised.

Approximately 50 million people have been infected with HIV worldwide. About half are men and there is now considerable epidemiological evidence to show that male circumcision gives significant protection against this disease. The most dramatic new evidence comes from Uganda, where heterosexual couples, in which the woman was HIV positive and her male partner was not, were studied over a 30-month period. The health team told both groups how to avoid infection and distributed free condoms, which 89 per cent of the men never bothered to use. At the end of the survey there had been no infections in any of the 50 circumcised men whilst 40 of the 137 uncircumcised had become HIV positive.[21] If males had never been circumcised I doubt if anyone in the medical establishment today would have thought that the operation might prove a useful tool in the fight against HIV/AIDS. We should bear this in mind before dismissing ancient practices and remedies out of hand.

One of the oldest religious practices is that of the pilgrimage: a journey, which in Old Testament times, the Israelites used to undertake three times a year to the central shrine, initially where the Ark was kept at Shiloh and later to Jerusalem.[22] For centuries people from all cultures have set out on these special expeditions full of hopes, and thankfulness, for healing and salvation. Such a long-standing worldwide custom must reflect a need in the human condition and the extent to which these needs are met will be considered next.

Chapter Three
Pilgrimages and their Healing Role

Pilgrimage is a journey to a spiritually charged centre. The journey may be easy or hazardous, sombre or festive, short or long, but whatever its outward form it is an important institution in all the world religions. The oldest pilgrimage is the *Kumbh Mela*. This takes place every twelve years and attracts millions of Hindus to the confluence of the sacred rivers in northern India, because they believe that bathing in these waters during the *Kumbh Mela* will help to heal and purify the body and the soul. For Muslims the most important pilgrimage is the *hajj*, this journey to the *Al-Ka'bah* (the House of Allah) in Mecca is one that all adult Muslims should undertake at least once in their lifetime, if they can afford it. These pilgrimages have a particularly high profile, but there are thousands of other centres to which people are drawn where they feel closer to their maker, and the urge to visit them is as strong now as it ever was, possibly because so much of life seems materialistic. Particularly compelling are those places, such as Lourdes, where the divine has apparently quite recently made contact with humanity.

Lourdes, a town situated in the French Pyrenees, is the most famous healing shrine in Europe. Here, according to Catholic teaching, the Virgin Mary appeared in a series of visions to a fourteen-year-old-girl, Marie Bernarde Soubirous, later canonized as Saint Bernadette. The Virgin told the child to wash in the spring and to arrange for a chapel to be built nearby: she was also to tell visitors to repent of their sins, to walk in processions, and to wash in and drink the waters. At the time, there was no sign of a spring and the Virgin did not say the sick would be healed by its waters.

Sightings of Mary had been reported near Lourdes for centuries, so Bernadette's visions were hardly unusual. There was, however, a special quality about them that, combined with the sudden appearance of a spring, captured the imagination of the faithful, first a few, and then increasing numbers, until Lourdes became a magnet attracting pilgrims from all parts of the world. About five million people visit Lourdes each year and of these about 10 per cent do so specifically for healing.[1]

Going to Lourdes

There is a saying, 'Rome is the head of the Church but Lourdes is its heart':
this expresses both the importance of Lourdes to the Catholic community
and the emotive overtones associated with the town and what it has to
offer. It also points to the sharp contrast that exists between the urban mas-
culinity of Rome and the rural feminine nature of Lourdes. Rome
represents leadership and authority, whilst Lourdes is more about the
'emotional side of Catholicism': it is the place where the sick and the suffering go in search of healing.[2]

A pilgrimage to Lourdes is an annual event for many Catholic dioceses
in Western Europe. Pilgrims travel by rail, coach and aeroplane, and a high
proportion are very ill people needing special care on the journey and during their stay. Among them, in 1985, was a patient we had admitted to St
Mary's Hospice with an inoperable brain tumour. He was stuporose and
had a short life expectancy, but made a good temporary recovery with
steroids. I was then asked to certify him as fit to travel to Lourdes. He had
visited the shrine for over twenty years, helping the sick as a *brancardier* (a
voluntary helper) and on this occasion he was to receive a papal medal for
long and meritorious service. All the arrangements had been made and I
can still remember his pleasure when he learnt he was going to Lourdes
that Saturday as a registered sick pilgrim. He had a wonderful time,
received his medal and died in the hospice about ten weeks later.

In a pilgrimage of 1,500 people there are likely to be 105 hospitalized
sick patients, who travel together as a group. Their constant care is provided by lay helpers supported by doctors and nurses. Before they set out, the
sick naturally experience some apprehension about what lies ahead, and
the journey is not likely to be comfortable or easy, but they adapt and, to
quote Dahlberg, are soon 'moved from the margins of secular society to
become the centre of a temporary community travelling towards the
sacred'.[3]

If you ask pilgrims who go to Lourdes regularly why they do so, you will
get similar answers from the healthy, the *brancardiers* and the sick pilgrims.
Their first visit had followed a bereavement, illness or tragedy and they had
found such meaning in the experience that once a pattern had been established they continued to go. Some find it almost addictive. The cures
associated with Lourdes are not highlighted by the ecclesiastical authorities. In fact, the reverse is true: the Church tends to be dismissive about
such events and emphasizes instead the spiritual fruits of the pilgrimage.
According to one guidebook, there are two healing springs at Lourdes –
the one uncovered by Bernadette, the other the Church's own spring,
which 'consists of the sacraments of Reconciliation, the new Baptism, and
the Eucharist, the food of eternal life'.[4] Pilgrims are constantly reminded of

the spiritual benefits to be attained through bodily suffering and of the primacy of the soul over the body. This is a traditional teaching of the Church that has a place in 'Ascetical Theology', but it can encourage an unhealthy sado-masochistic attitude to pain when it would be kinder to remove it. I am mindful, for instance, of being asked to visit a nun in hospital who had disseminated breast cancer and was being encouraged, by her confessor, to use the pain as a means of gaining spiritual grace. This is acceptable if nothing can be done to ease the pain, but luckily the senior nurse, who was also a nun, disapproved of this approach and insisted that I should be consulted so that her patient's distress could be relieved.

Handicapped Children at Lourdes

Some pilgrimages to Lourdes cater for people with special needs: the Handicapped Children's Pilgrimage is one of these. It is organized by a charitable trust which raises all the funds needed for the children's journey, whilst expecting the helpers to pay their own expenses. Each year about 4,000 children go to Lourdes under this scheme, together with their helpers, nurses, priests and doctors: it is a remarkable gathering of people who, for the most part, have never met before setting out together. The children may be physically or mentally handicapped, blind, epileptic or deaf; the group may also include children with autism, leukaemia, spina bifida or cerebral palsy. Their helpers are mainly young Catholics who regard themselves as 'pilgrims who help the sick'.

Dahlberg accompanied one such pilgrimage and speaks of the carnival-like atmosphere that he experienced. Every child has its own helper, usually someone below the age of thirty, and they all stay in the same hotel in Lourdes. The children are not regarded as sick but as handicapped and each morning begins with the helpers, who are mostly untrained, bathing and dressing the children and helping them with their breakfast. This constant commitment makes heavy physical and mental demands on the volunteers and some have only two or three hours' sleep a night, but the children have a great holiday.

The focus is not on the hope of a miraculous cure but on the loving care of the suffering body. The possibility of a cure occurring at the shrine is discussed, but this is not something the children are encouraged to anticipate; the guidebook they use stresses that the expectation of a miracle is not the purpose of the pilgrimage. The children are encouraged to bear their afflictions cheerfully because this enables them to acquire the grace that will make them Christ-like. The real miracle, they are told, is the forgiveness of sin and great emphasis is placed on the expiatory role of physical suffering and its creative function.[5]

At Lourdes, sick people are seen as very special and are accorded an unusual sanctity vis-à-vis the healthy visitors. Other pilgrims treat them almost like saints, asking for their prayers, approaching and touching them and offering them small gifts. They are, as a matter of course, accorded favoured treatment at the religious ceremonies held at the basilicas and within the town. They are a special category in a special place, and other pilgrims are naturally moved 'to pray for healing for everyone and especially for the sick'.[6]

The Sick at Lourdes

A focal point in Lourdes is the spring that was revealed to Bernadette; it currently produces 20,000 gallons of water a week. The spring soon became associated with miraculous cures and its water is available both for drinking and immersion: there are special bathhouses for those who wish to bathe. Only a small number, about 9 per cent, visit the baths, and most of these are female. Bathing at Lourdes is carefully organized by the *brancardiers* or, in the female section, by volunteers called *handmaids*. Anyone may bathe, but sick pilgrims are always given priority and are immersed as quickly as possible. Inside the bathhouse, pilgrims are directed into cubicles where they strip to their underclothes and then proceed to the bathing area. The *brancardiers* now take them behind a curtain, where the pilgrims remove their underclothes and cover themselves with a damp towel, before being helped into the waters. The waters are bitterly cold, so after only a few moments' immersion the bathers return to their cubicles. Pilgrims never dry themselves before they dress again, but everyone says that the body dries remarkably quickly. This brief description deals only with the commonplace physical aspects of the process: perhaps more important, but impossible to put into words, are the prayers, expectations and devotional attitude of both the attendants and the bathers themselves.

As most people believe that it is in the baths that the sick will be healed, bathing them can be a profound experience for the *brancardiers* and *handmaids*. This applies particularly when the individual is obviously very ill and willingly accepts the major ordeal that immersion in cold water can be. But this possibility is now played down by the Church authorities; instead, they draw parallels with the sacrament of baptism and see the immersion as symbolizing membership of the Church, purgation of sins, Christ's sacrificial act and His resurrection from the dead. Despite this official attitude, people continue to enter the baths in the hope of being cured or obtaining relief from personal problems. Some sick pilgrims, supported by their helpers, movingly cry aloud to be cured during the bathing, and there are times when the atmosphere can become quite tense.[7]

The Lourdes experience is not limited to bathing in the grotto. Magnificent processions are held daily on the esplanade, a large open space in front of the basilicas where people from all over the world mingle together. The most important procession is that of the Blessed Sacrament when the officiating bishop blesses the sick with a monstrance, a cross holding the consecrated host. Immediately behind the bishop and leading the rest of the procession come the visiting doctors; they may be of any religious persuasion and not necessarily Catholic.[8] Huge torch-lit processions are held at night: these are profoundly moving spectacles and remarkably quiet, except when the crowds sing the Lourdes hymn. Some processions provide an opportunity for different groups of pilgrims to parade with their national flags and the banners of their local region and diocese. These colourful occasions tend to emphasize the community of all believers and are not particularly concerned with cures, but if someone does claim to be healed during the procession, the *brancardiers* are instructed to remove that person immediately from the esplanade and take them to the Medical Bureau for assessment.[9]

Criteria for Assessing Claims at Lourdes

Many people believe that they have been healed at Lourdes and the evidence that cures do take place is well documented, but the number of claims of miraculous healing that are accepted as such is small – only sixty-seven since 1868. All such claims are examined with great care. The Catholic Church has much experience in dealing with claimed miracles and the criteria it uses at Lourdes are based on principles laid down in 1735 by Cardinal Lambertini, who later became Pope Benedict XIV. They are as follows:

- The diagnosis has to be established by medically qualified doctors.
- The illness has to be a physical one; cures of mental illness are not accepted as miraculous.
- The disease has to have advanced to the point where it is incurable.
- The cure has to be instantaneous (this was later amended to include cures occurring over a few days).
- The cure has to be complete and permanent.
- No treatment should have been given that might have facilitated the cure.
- The person claiming the cure has to be a registered sick pilgrim and possess the relevant medical documents; these must have been completed before the pilgrimage began. This requirement has a twofold purpose. It enables the doctors and nurses accompanying the pilgrimage to have the information they need to provide appropriate care for the sick. It also helps to eliminate any unjustified claims of being healed.

A claim for a miraculous cure has to pass four separate hurdles before it is accepted as valid. These are the Medical Bureau, the International Medical Committee of Lourdes, the Bishop's Canonical Commission and final approval has to be given by the Diocesan Bishop himself.

The Medical Assessment

It is members of the Medical Bureau who first look into claims of miraculous cures. This was established in 1883 by Baron de St Maclou, a physician, and it welcomes any doctor who wishes to participate in its work. It is located in Lourdes and anyone who claims to have been cured must contact the Medical Bureau and produce medical documents to support their claim. If the evidence seems reasonable, the Bureau opens a dossier for that patient and invites her – most patients are female – to return the following year. The president of the Bureau next contacts the patient's doctors for further details and collates all the available information: this is examined by all interested doctors when the patient returns for review. At this stage the claim may be rejected or a decision taken to review the case annually for at least two more years. Some may then be referred to the next stage of the process, assessment by the International Medical Committee of Lourdes (CMIL).

The CMIL is a committee of thirty Catholic doctors who meet annually in Paris to examine cases referred to them by the Medical Bureau. They are nominated by the bishops and chosen from a wide range of specialities: most live in countries that send regular pilgrimages to Lourdes. If the CMIL decides that a claim merits further investigation, it asks one of its members to examine the background in greater detail and provide a written report. This is carefully discussed under eighteen headings, with a vote being taken at each stage. In its discussions the committee is expected to cover the criteria laid down by Cardinal Lambertini. It then decides whether the follow-up period has been sufficient to ensure that the disease will not recur, and finally answer the question, 'Does the cure of this person constitute a phenomenon which is contrary to the observations and expectations of medical knowledge and scientifically inexplicable?' If the answer is 'yes', the patient's bishop is notified: he will then refer the subject to his Canonical Commission before deciding if the cure can be declared miraculous.[10] Such an outcome is very rare.

Between 1947 and 1977 about 120 million pilgrims visited Lourdes. Many of these approached the Medical Bureau believing that they had been cured, but only 30,000 were invited to return for review the following year of whom only fifty-five were referred to the CMIL. At the end of the consultation process just twenty-seven people were considered to have had a cure for which there was no medical explanation, and of these only thirteen were regarded as miraculous cures.[11] One was Delizia Cirolli, a Sicilian girl who was declared to be inexplicably cured of a Ewing's tumour by the CMIL in 1982 and, a few years later, adjudged to have been miraculously cured.

Delizia's story begins in 1976 when she was twelve years old and found to have a tumour of the right knee, which was diagnosed initially as a bony metastasis of a neuroblastoma. The orthopaedic surgeon wanted to amputate the leg but the parents rejected his advice and took Delizia to Lourdes. Despite bathing in the water, praying and attending the ceremonies, her condition continued to deteriorate and her mother began to prepare for Delizia's funeral. At the same time the villagers continued to pray to Our Lady of Lourdes on her behalf and her mother continued to give her Lourdes water at home. Four months later, shortly before Christmas, Delizia said that she wanted to get up and go outside, which she did without pain, though she was still very weak and weighed only 22 kg. Her general health improved, the swelling of the knee subsided and she was reassessed by the Medical Bureau at Lourdes for the next four years. Her case was then sent to the CMIL, which declared her inexplicably cured in September 1982. Although the initial diagnosis was of a neuroblastoma, and this remains plausible, subsequent review by eminent histologists favoured the diagnosis of a Ewing's sarcoma. Spontaneous remission of a neuroblastoma has been reported very rarely and never after the age of five. There is no record of a spontaneous remission of a Ewing's tumour.[12]

The Effect of Pilgrimage on Anxiety and Depression

When people go to Lourdes and claim to have been cured, their claim is investigated only if they were suffering from a physical disease. People with psychiatric illnesses cannot be classified as miraculously cured, yet many people visit Lourdes in the hope that their mental distress will be eased. Despite the prevalence of such distress no one studied changes in the psychological well-being of pilgrims until Morris did so in 1982.[13]

Morris's study was designed to determine whether a pilgrimage to Lourdes would reduce levels of anxiety and depression or alter the depth of a person's religious belief. For this purpose he used three questionnaires: the State-Tait Anxiety Inventory, the Beck Depression Inventory and the Religious Attitude Scale of Poppleton and Pilkington. He invited fifty elderly people who were scheduled to go on a diocesan pilgrimage as registered sick pilgrims to take part in the survey. He later rejected two pilgrims because of severe dementia, and twenty-two refused to participate mainly because they felt that they were too ill, too old or just too frightened to undergo repeated psychological assessments. Some members of this group in fact died or were hospitalized before the pilgrimage began.

Twenty-six patients remained in his study group. Their average age was sixty, and the group included people with cancer, leukaemia, muscular dystrophy, ulcerative colitis, spastic diplegia, spinal injury, multiple sclerosis and brain damage.

They did not feel physically better after the visit. They did, however, consider that the pilgrimage had been worthwhile, and that it had strengthened their religious faith, made them more relaxed and more content, and better able to accept their physical disabilities. The psychological tests revealed a considerable reduction in anxiety ($p = 0.01$) and depression ($p = 0.01$) on their return from Lourdes, and this improvement was maintained during the following year. The quality of life of most of the pilgrims was improved by their visit and Morris suggests that pilgrimage might be worth considering for other chronically sick people with a religious frame of mind who have difficulty in accepting their condition.

Padre Pio and San Giovanni Rotondo

It is axiomatic that a pilgrimage is a journey to a sacred place which lies beyond the mundane realm of the pilgrim's daily experience.[14] However, some places attract pilgrims not because the site has any special religious significance but because of the spiritual stature of a person living there. This was the case with San Giovanni Rotondo, an obscure village in southern Italy, where the Capuchin Friar Padre Pio dwelt for many years. It now attracts more than seven million visitors a year, surpassing Lourdes in popularity and second only to the site dedicated to Our Lady of Guadalupe in Mexico.

Padre Pio was born in 1887 in Pietrelcina. The son of a poor peasant family, he was a pious child who entered the Capuchin novitiate at the age of sixteen and became a priest in 1910. At that time, the Capuchin order was noted for its austerity and the fact that all its friars were bearded was a sign of their ascetic lifestyle. The rigour of the Capuchin order suited Pio's spiritual temperament, but the deprivations often made him ill and he was once sent home because his superiors thought he might die. Later, in 1916, he was sent to the small friary at San Giovanni Rotondo where, it was hoped, he might benefit from the mountain air. His health did improve and, except for a few months, he remained there until his death.

Once established in the friary, Pio undertook the spiritual direction of members of the local community and soon became known in the area as a holy friar. On 20 September 1918, whilst praying in the friary church, he had a vision which he described, in a letter to his confessor, in these words. 'There appeared before me a man whose hands and feet and side were dripping with blood and when the vision disappeared I realized that my own hands, feet and side were bleeding.' News of the stigmatization spread rapidly and people began travelling to San Giovanni Rotondo to seek a 'grace', such as a cure or other favour, from this holy man.[15] He was to attract an enormous popular following.

Among those who visited him much later was a lady I cared for briefly during her terminal illness. She was a tertiary of the Servite order and had attended Padre Pio's mass when, quite unexpectedly, members of her party were invited to meet the father. He removed his mittens before walking past them and the stigmata on his wrists and feet were clearly visible. These had been examined by a surgeon, Professor Francesco di Raimondo, who had found them to be 'medically inexplicable'.

Padre Pio was the first Catholic priest to bear the stigmata. He died in 1968, was beatified on 2 March 1999 and canonized on 16 June 2002. He is associated with many healing miracles and charitable works, but his main concern was the cure of souls and he spent many hours in prayer and in the confessional helping people, almost invariably men, with their spiritual problems. He was also concerned with people's physical well-being and supported projects to drain mosquito-infested swamps and improve local medical facilities. One of his most visible achievements was the building of a 500-bed hospital, which attracted leading cardiologists from all over the world to San Giovanni Rotondo.

I have personal knowledge of one of the miracles attributed to Padre Pio as it involved my friend John Mitchell. John's condition was desperate when I sent him to hospital for an emergency operation. Initially, he made a good post-operative recovery but then he relapsed and his condition rapidly worsened. For days he had almost unbearable abdominal pain, and lay awake at night watching the ward clock tick away the seconds, unable to sleep because of the intense pain. The night when his family had been warned to expect his death, he had a vision. He remembers the precise time it appeared: it was exactly five o'clock when the Friar stood beside his bed. His face was hidden by a cowl and he wore the long habit of his order with girdle and rosary. John knew instinctively that it was Padre Pio and at the same time he felt an indescribable sense of bliss and peace. He went into a deep sleep and the next morning was free from pain. During the night a large amount of foul smelling fluid had discharged through the wound in his abdominal wall. He is convinced that Padre Pio visited him, even though Pio had been dead for some years and the healing took place in a hospital in England.

Jerusalem

Jerusalem is one of the great centres of pilgrimage, and it is easy to understand why it is the focus of so much religious devotion and fervour. It contains within a small compass the most sacred places of Judaism, Christianity and, after Mecca and Medina, of Islam. Here Jews meet and pray at the Western Wall on the site of Solomon's temple; Christians follow the route Jesus took along the Via Dolorosa when he carried his cross to Golgotha and gaze into the garden tomb where he may have been laid after the crucifixion: and Muslims can visit the Dome of the Rock, which enshrines the place where Muhammad ascended to heaven on the *Al-Miraj*. The very stones of the city act as a magnet to Christians, Jews and Muslims alike, yet strangely it is not reputed to be a 'healing centre' in the way that Lourdes is.

An outstanding characteristic of Jerusalem is the wide variety of people and cultures found there. The Old City has Jewish, Christian, Armenian and Muslim quarters and within the city there are twenty-seven distinct Christian communities which regularly arrange pilgrimages to the Holy Land. The expectations of any particular pilgrim group is likely to depend on their religious tradition. Those of Greek Orthodox Christians, for instance, are likely to differ considerably from those of American Protestants or of Messianic Jews.

Greek Orthodox pilgrims are most likely to visit the Holy Land in their old age, to prepare themselves for a good death and for their subsequent acceptance into heaven. Their pilgrimage involves two types of activity. The first is concerned with 'the transformation of the fallen into the redeemed', the second focuses on 'collective participation', a sense of being united with all other Orthodox Christians. The transformation of the fallen into the redeemed has three stages: the first takes place in the pilgrims' homeland, before they set out on their journey, when they unburden their souls by the act of sacramental confession. The second stage is the washing of feet when they enter the Holy Land. This is done at the port of entry by monks of the Brotherhood of the Holy Sepulchre: it symbolizes the replacement of worldly interests whilst maintaining their normal duties to family and neighbours, by a closer pursuit of eternal realities. Third, they are baptized like Christ in the River Jordan with the expectation that the Holy Spirit will descend upon them and renew them.

The second aspect of an Orthodox pilgrimage, which focuses on 'collective participation', reaches its culmination during Holy Week which they observe in Jerusalem. The atmosphere of goodwill is then so tangible that they witness more clearly than ever before the reality of the community united in Christ. There is an easy warmth in their relationship with strangers which they feel unable to express in their normal social life. This is most movingly expressed as they celebrate the Orthodox Liturgy and announce the imminence of the resurrection by passing the Holy Fire from hand to hand until the entire church is ablaze with the flames of thousands of 'resurrection candles'; and again, later in the day, as they prepare to break the Lenten fast and sing together the hymn 'Christ is risen from the dead', *Christos Anesti*.[16]

Eastern Orthodox pilgrims long to be healed physically as well as spiritually. This was made clear to me by Canon Andrew White of Coventry Cathedral, who was present when the Anglican Bishops of Coventry and Nigeria met the Syrian Orthodox Archbishop of Jerusalem on 8 January 2001 to sign an agreement of mutual support. This ceremony was held in St Mark's monastery and church, the oldest church in Christendom, and reputedly the place where Jesus and the disciples met for the Last Supper. During the ceremony, Bishop Josiah of Nigeria had a severe bout of malaria and his temperature rose to 41°C. The monks took him to a room reserved for the sick and after studying their ancient medical books treated him with a mixture of arrack and garlic. They assured the dignitaries that there was no need to worry about Bishop Josiah as the church was the house of miracles and they were used to caring for the sick: the bishop recovered.

People visit the monks every week for healing and the large pile of crutches left in the church is a testimony of their success rate. An English clergyman, in a recent letter to a member of the monastic community, claimed to have been completely healed of cancer at St Mark's.

Protestants who visit the Holy Land also like to be baptized in the River Jordan. I witnessed such a ceremony when I visited in 1998. It was a very evocative scene, which struck a hidden chord within the psyche. I remember that the water was very cold and that the participants, all Americans, were wearing white robes. Those who had been baptized previously were renewing their vows, but some were being immersed for the first time.

I have many vivid recollections of my visit to Jerusalem and among these is a visit to St John's Ophthalmic Hospital where so much good work is done for the Palestinians. I was disappointed with the Via Dolorosa, the path Jesus took to Calvary. It was much shorter than I expected and we were given little time by our Israeli guide to absorb the atmosphere and contemplate its significance. I can understand now why Catholic pilgrims who have meditated deeply on the Stations of the Cross at home sometimes prefer to proceed along the Via Dolorosa with their eyes downcast, even closed, so that the physical reality of what they might see does not blur the inner reality on which they focus in their meditations. For the most part they are seeking a more profound awareness of the presence of Christ as well as spiritual renewal.

It would be wrong to emphasize any great distinction between the goals of a Catholic and an Orthodox pilgrimage, but it may be true to say that

Orthodox pilgrims hope for a transfiguration that will prepare them for the 'world to come' whilst Catholic pilgrims are more concerned with renewal, and a recharging of the spiritual energies that have been drained by involvement with the secular world: they seek to be repossessed by the Spirit that inspires and gives meaning to their life and labours. Protestant pilgrims to the Holy Land will experience a similar longing for renewal but they also welcome the opportunity to relate the archaeological sites more closely with the events recorded in the Bible.

One of the sites that Protestant Christians own, and like to visit, is the Garden Tomb in Jerusalem. This is a careful reconstruction of a rich man's garden in the style of the first century CE which contains a tomb that many believe is the actual site of Christ's burial. Christians like to hold a Holy Communion service there and I was fortunate to attend one that was con-celebrated by an Anglican and a Catholic priest. There were, possibly, Christian Zionists among the other groups holding services in the garden while we were there, but they would have been following a completely different agenda.

Christian Zionists are a small but active group of biblical fundamentalists. They believe that they have the divinely ordained task of bringing about Christ's Second Coming and of helping to destroy the forces of evil. They also believe they have to encourage Jews in the Diaspora to return to the Promised Land and that this will lead to the re-establishment of the Solomonic Temple and its ordained rituals. On their annual Feast of the Tabernacles pilgrimage Christian Zionists seek to comfort the Jews and further the work of God. Much of their time is spent listening to lectures by Israeli politicians and by a pressure group called the International Christian Embassy. The talks are interspersed with regular prayer meetings and guided tours of the surrounding areas. These include visits to religious schools where Orthodox Jews are taught to perform the rituals of sacrifice so that they will be ready for the moment when the Temple is rebuilt and stands once again on the site now occupied by the Al-Aqsa mosque and the Dome of the Rock. There are healing sessions throughout the week but the highlight for these pilgrims is a 'Praise Procession' when they march along the route that the Messiah will take when he returns to earth, waving banners and palms, and singing the praises of Israel and of the imminence of Christ's return.[17]

Jerusalem is not only a centre of Christian pilgrimage. It attracts people of many beliefs most especially Muslims and Jews. Jerusalem has always been the centre of aspiration for the Jewish people and represents more than just a Holy City; it is the capital of the Promised Land, the country that God pledged to Abraham and his descendants forever. Some believe that this promise is about to be realized as more and more Jews return to their homeland, Israel. Increasingly, there is the expectation that the

Temple will be rebuilt, that the Messiah will soon appear and all other nations will then have to recognize the pre-eminent position of Jews as God's Chosen People.

It was from Jerusalem that the Prophet Muhammad made his famous night journey to paradise, where he is said to have met and talked with the prophets who had preceded him, including Moses and Jesus, and to have been granted an ineffable Vision of God. The *Al-Miraj* was probably part of the vision, but later accounts made it into an actual journey astride the winged horse Buraq. The site of the ascension is marked by the Dome of the Rock, a famous attraction for pilgrims and tourists alike. There are always tensions where conflicting streams of religious fervour coalesce but nowhere is this so apparent as in Jerusalem.

Healing and Pilgrimage in Sri Lanka

The superficial beauty of Sri Lanka cannot hide completely the culture of violence that has disrupted life on the island since 1983. The Tamil Tigers waged a war of attrition on the central government for many years and the country has one of the highest suicide rates in the world, but religious practices seem relatively untroubled by such trauma. The population is predominantly Buddhist though there are large Hindu and Muslim minorities; only 7 per cent are practising Christians. Given these figures it is not surprising that the main centre of pilgrimage is a Buddhist one. The shrine of Kataragama attracts hundreds of thousands of pilgrims a year, not because there is any historical association with the Buddha but because people believe that their prayers will be answered there. This is a powerful inducement to devotion. Whatever the troubles that afflict them, the god Kataragama will 'deliver the goods'.[18]

Sri Lankan Christians are mainly Catholics. They have their own healing shrines and the most popular ones, before the country gained independence in 1948, were at St Anne's in Talawila and the church at Madhu. Miraculous cures were claimed at both shrines with St Anne's being especially noted for 'healing people who were possessed'. Bishop Joudain of Ceylon commenting on this wrote: 'it would appear that St Anne's has a very special power over the devil'. Supplicants are not bathed in water at these shrines; their treatment is more unusual, even bizarre: they are buried up to the neck in the sand that fronts the churches, or tied to crosses with their hands extended above their heads.

For socio-political reasons the importance of these shrines declined after the country became a republic and people now tend to visit them on a 'day out' rather than for any therapeutic or spiritual reason. The most significant feature of both shrines is the sand. Even today, just as pilgrims to Lourdes and Knock take bottles of holy water home with them for the sick, so the Sri Lankans take sand from the vicinity of these shrines. At Talawila they collect it from around the church: at Madhu they scoop it from a hole in the church floor, the sand being replaced during the major festivals.[19]

The shrines at Talawila and Madhu are 'space-centred'; in other words, they derive their importance from the location in which they are set. The new shrines that have replaced them are 'person-centred' and, as with Padre Pio at San Giovanni, derive their significance from the person associated with them. One such shrine is at Suvagama. This is centred on Brother Lambert, who is considered to have a special relationship with the Virgin Mary. He wanted to become a priest, but his family was too poor to finance his training so he had to undertake low-paid, boring jobs. Then he had dreams and visions of the Virgin Mary who told him that he had been chosen for a special task – to heal the sick – and she gave him a miraculous rosary, which is effective only in his hands. His healing ministry has been so successful that he attracts hundreds of people to his services each weekend.

The focal character at the shrine devoted to Our Lady of Kutanayake is a man who calls himself Bishop Aponsu. He also wished to be a priest but failed to complete his studies at the seminary. Aponsu carries the marks of the stigmata and claims to have been ordained by Christ himself. Many people believe that he possesses divine powers and that he is equally effective at healing their physical and mental problems. Not surprisingly, he has a large following who attend his weekly rituals. As with Brother Lambert, his healing ability is seen as a personal talent and is not regarded as being related to the shrine itself.

It is not just the sick who flock to these healers, nor are the pilgrims mainly impoverished peasants or fishermen. The shrines attract people from the towns and the middle classes, people who are not seeking spiritual blessings but help in getting a job, recovering stolen property and countering sorcery. Sorcery has a high profile in modern Sri Lanka and whilst misfortune was once attributed to demonic forces, it now tends to be seen as the work of sorcerers acting on behalf of clients. It is fear of sorcery that drives most people to these new Catholic shrines; once people looked to the priest for protection against the works of the devil but now he is seen as powerless, and this role of his has been invested in the holy man.[20]

Pilgrimages and Healing in Islam

Pilgrimage is one of the 'Five Pillars of Islam', the five duties incumbent upon a Muslim. The first is to recite the *Shahada*, the profession of faith – 'There is no God but God, Muhammad is the Messenger of God' – in public.

Merely by repeating these words with conviction and understanding, one becomes a Muslim. The second requirement is the observance of prayer (*salat*); this should be done five times a day either alone or in congregation behind an imam. The third is the payment of legal alms (*zakat*), the fourth is to keep the annual fast (*thaum*) during Ramadhan and the fifth is the pilgrimage to Mecca.

There are many centres of pilgrimage in the Islamic world but Mecca, the birthplace of Muhammad, is the most important and the annual pilgrimage to Mecca, the *hajj*, must be undertaken at least once in the lifetime by every Muslim who can afford it. It symbolizes the unity of humanity and is a time when Muslims from all parts of the world meet as equals to worship Allah: in doing so we are told that they experience a unique sense of being in the presence of their Creator.[21] Medina and Jerusalem are the other most important pilgrim centres, but Muslims visit many other shrines. Some, like Kota in Kashmir, are 'person-centred', whilst among the 'space-centred' ones is the Ummayad Mosque in Damascus. This mosque contains the mausoleum of John the Baptist, revered in Islam as the Prophet Yahya and regarded by Muslims as the fourth most holy place in the world.[22]

About three million Muslims undertake the *hajj* each year. The pilgrimage rite begins on the seventh day of *Dhul Hijjah*, the twelfth month of the Islamic calendar, and ends on the twelfth day, so there is a massive influx of people into Mecca during a very short time. All pilgrims wear the garments of Ihram – two seamless white sheets wrapped around the body, as an outer sign that they have entered an inner state of holiness and purity. In Mecca they walk seven times around the sacred Ka'bah in the Great Mosque, kiss or touch the black stone in the Ka'bah, pray towards the Ka'bah and the sacred stone, the *Maqam Ibrahim*, and then run seven times between the points known as Mount Safa and Mount Marwah. Between the eighth and twelfth days of *Dhul Hijjah* they visit the holy places outside Mecca and sacrifice an animal to commemorate Abraham's sacrifice of a ram. Then their heads are shaved and they throw stones at pillars, which represent devils. The last rite of the pilgrimage is the farewell *tawaf*, the encircling of the Ka'bah, before they leave the city.

Muslims who live in Mecca and others who do not feel ready for the *hajj* undertake a minor pilgrimage called the *'umrah*. This also begins with donning the garments of Ihram – assuming the state of ritual purity – and with a declaration of intent (*niyah*) to perform the *'umrah*. The pilgrim walks around the Ka'bah seven times, touches the black stone, prays at the *Maqam Ibrahim*, drinks the water of the sacred Zamzam well, touches the black stone again, runs seven times between Mount Safa and Mount Marwah, and completes the *'umrah* by shaving the head.

I do not know whether those completing the *hajj* or *'umrah* receive individual healing, but the focus on purification, and a general accord with the

rest of Islam, must be uplifting despite the hardships involved, and is probably, in the widest sense of the term, a source of healing. Perhaps the lack
of emphasis on this aspect of pilgrimage may be related to the almost complete absence of healing miracles in the Qu'rān. Only one comes to mind:
it is in Sūrah 12, which relates the story of Joseph (Yūsaf) and tells how
Jacob became blind when he was told of his son's death, and regained his
sight when he learnt that he was still alive.

> And he [Jacob] turned away from them,
> And said, 'How great
> Is my grief for Joseph!'
> And his eyes became white
> With sorrow, and he fell
> Into silent melancholy. (verse 84)

> Then when the bearer
> Of the good news came,
> He cast [the shirt]
> Over his face, and he
> Forthwith regained clear sight. (verse 96)[23]

Muslims say that there are two types of miracles: ordinary daily miracles
and the miracles God uses to change the direction of events. Like
Christians, they also distinguish between living saints and dead saints and
make pilgrimages to the shrines of both. Their living saints are likely to be
involved in specific social activities, for example caring for the poor and
providing them with food and clothing. One centre in Kashmir is famous
for its care of abandoned children, looking after them until the boys can
find employment and the girls suitable marriages. Hundreds of thousands
of pilgrims visit centres such as this.

Muslims often regard a pilgrimage as an outing, a 'day out' in which
people put on their best clothes and have a good time, but they also realize that it must have a more serious theme and during the pilgrimage will
pray for some special grace such as a personal healing or the recovery from
illness of a close relative or friend. Some Sufi centres have healing services:
these often have a charismatic aspect, similar to Pentecostal ones. Those
who receive healing are not left isolated afterwards, but are given continuing support and a programme of prayer and meditation for their comfort.

One cautionary note needs to be sounded, however. Pilgrimages are
never without some element of danger and the extreme overcrowding and
oppressive heat encountered on the *hajj* poses considerable health risks to
pilgrims, most significantly that of meningitis. Although the risk of infection with Meningitis A and C is well recognized, a new strain (W135
meningococcal disease) emerged as a major hazard of the *hajj* in 2000.

Over the following two years, seventy-nine cases of W135 meningococcal disease occurred in Muslim pilgrims returning to the UK, and of these eighteen died.[24] Since that outbreak the government of Saudi Arabia has made quadrivalent meningococcal vaccination (ACWY Vac) a visa require-ment for pilgrims whilst the UK government now provides leaflets for its Muslim community, giving appropriate advice in six languages.

African Centres

Africa is a vast continent in which there is great religious and cultural diver-sity. The most sophisticated medical centres coexist with the continued practice of tribal medicine by witch doctors, and it is not surprising that there is a marked difference in the attitude to illness in these two compet-ing cultures. In contrast to the scientific approach of Western medicine, many Africans are likely to blame their illness on sorcery or malevolent spirits, and they seek to counter these with the help of witch doctors and the ancestors. Within this tradition there are many groves, rivers and mountains that are considered sacred: these are places where nature spir-its dwell, where the ancestors can be contacted and the sick healed. One such place is the Motouleng fertility cave in South Africa.

The Motouleng cave has been a place of pilgrimage for Africans for cen-turies. It has been described as the African version of Lourdes and is one of South Africa's most sacred sites. Thousands of people visit the cave for healing and support, drawn by the ancestral spirits that, tradition says, inhabit the cave. Motouleng is one of the largest caves in the Southern hemisphere and its interior is constantly lit by coloured candles, which flicker on rough stone altars where gifts are placed as an offering to the ancestral spirits. A traditional healer, Gladys Dlamini, lives in a cave close by. She says that many miracles take place at Motouleng, that she herself can cure the blind and the disabled with magic herbs, and that the spirits tell her which herbs to use.[25]

Unfortunately, Motouleng is no longer the peaceful place it once was. In recent years there has been increasing conflict between the owners of the neighbouring properties and visitors to the cave. This follows an attempt by the former to restrict access to the site and there has been violence and bloodshed as a result. Motouleng is not alone in this respect; worse dis-putes occur daily in Jerusalem, the focus of so many prayers for peace, reconciliation and goodwill.

There are many other healing centres in Africa but a visit to them can have bitter repercussions. I have in front of me a report from 'Ethiopiaid', dated November 1999. It tells the story of Miftah, a fourteen-year-old-boy who was lame from birth. His mother took him to a Christian place of pilgrimage in Ethiopia where there is a holy spring, which, it is claimed, can heal the sick. Miftah stayed there for two months but there was no improvement. His mother, a Muslim, was then rejected by her family for taking the boy to a Christian shrine, and in despair she fled and disappeared. Miftah then made his way to Addis Ababa where he worked as a shoeshine boy before being admitted to the Manageshe home for disabled children.[26]

Miftah's story illustrates the lengths to which people are prepared to go to find healing for themselves and those they love. Some have to bear the burden of disappointment if the search is unsuccessful; few are physically healed but most seem to derive some benefit from their pilgrimage. They often gain a sense of inner peace and a greater certainty of their ability to cope, and I have yet to meet a pilgrim who regrets having made the journey.

Healing at Glastonbury

Pilgrimages do not have to be to faraway places, they can be to local shrines and one that I attend annually is the pilgrimage to Glastonbury, the oldest Christian centre in England. Glastonbury is the focus of many historical allusions and myths including the legend that Joseph of Arimathea brought Jesus there on a trading expedition. It is also a New Age centre and the venue of the largest annual pop festival in the UK. It has two main physical features, the Tor, a conical hill visible for many miles across the Somerset Levels, and the ruined Abbey of St Mary. This was the most famous monastery in Britain until Henry VIII broke with the Catholic Church in 1529 and dissolved the monasteries. The abbey then fell into disrepair but since the 1950s there has been an annual pilgrimage to the ruins in July. These are happy, relaxed occasions when after celebrating the Holy Eucharist, children are free to play in the abbey grounds and family groups sit together to picnic.

Pilgrimages are often associated with miraculous cures, so it seems right to include here the story of my healing at Glastonbury. It was not a momentous event but it was my own and therefore special for me. It happened many years ago during the Eucharist. We were standing near the site of the original high altar, and separate from the main concourse of people and celebrants. I had forgotten to take my reading glasses but, quite unexpectedly, I found myself able to read the script on the service leaflet quite easily. This may not seem a big deal, particularly as I do not usually need an order of service when attending a Eucharist, but this was different: the script was small, parts of the service, including some hymns, were unfamiliar, and I had not been able to read without spectacles for years. My wife was aware of what was happening but did not mention it at the time in case she 'broke the spell'. This new clarity of vision was temporary: it lasted only during the service, and by the next day I needed spectacles to read as usual. I still cannot decide on a satisfactory explanation: sometimes I think it was just a trick of the light but I cannot help wondering if it might have been a small miracle.

I like to visit the Chalice Well gardens when I am in Glastonbury. This is a private trust property situated at the foot of the Tor and the grounds are most beautifully maintained. Many people regard it as a sacred site with a special affinity to Jesus, and it attracts people from many parts of the world, most noticeably young adults. They have come on what they regard as a pilgrimage to an important spiritual centre, and there they sit and meditate and enjoy the water that flows from the well within the gardens. This well is very old, probably pre-dating the Roman era, and never runs dry. The water is ice cold and is said to have healing properties. People wash in it, drink it and carry bottles of it away with them. It stains the skin a brownish colour so it probably contains high levels of iron, which would make it a most effective medicine for anyone with iron-deficiency anaemia.

Perhaps I should mention some other reasons why I personally am attracted to this area: my wife and I visited Glastonbury in 1952 on our honeymoon, my daughters attended a nearby school and my son-in-law lived in a house that once stood within the walls of the gardens.

Chapter Four
Judaeo-Christian Perspective

Healing has always been closely linked to people's religious practices and spiritual beliefs, and this remains true today when many are unsure of what they really believe. The connection is so consistent that it would be difficult to portray the history of healing without mentioning some of the miraculous events recorded in the Bible, and in particular the New Testament. The healings mentioned in the Old Testament are mainly associated with two critical periods in Jewish history – the Exodus led by Moses and the ministry of the prophets Elijah and Elisha[1] – but the first report of a healing goes back even further, to the time of Abraham and a King called Abimelech whose women were barren until Abraham interceded with God: 'and God healed Abimelech, his wife and his slave girls, and they bore children'.[2]

Another well-known example of group healing occurred when, after their escape from Egypt, the Jews were living in the desert and complained about the hardships they were enduring. God punished them for their grumbling and 'sent poisonous snakes among the people and many were bitten and died'. When Moses interceded with God, he was told to make a bronze serpent and place it on a pole so that anyone who looked at it would be healed of the snakebites. This story hints at a belief in the power of sympathetic magic, which holds that like cures like. Whatever the reason may be, the bronze serpent healed the sufferers and freed the Israelites from the plague of snakes.[3]

The same idea is evident in the Christian doctrine of vicarious suffering and redemption. This asserts that the sins of the whole world have been redeemed by the elevation of Christ on the Cross, and for the Christian believer this is the most perfect example of group healing. Here, in a single act, God in Christ freed the world of sin and conquered death forever.

The Widow's Son

The Old Testament contains two accounts of the healing of a widow's son. In one the healing is ascribed to Elijah,[4] in the other to the prophet Elisha.[5] The stories are very similar and describe the first successful resuscitation of a dead person by mouth-to-mouth respiration.

A young man died suddenly and his mother was numb with grief and angry with God and his prophet whom she had often helped. She sent for him and he came immediately. Both accounts say that the prophet prayed, possibly using an 'arrow prayer', a short, intense cry for help. He then breathed into the boy's mouth and restored him to life. The text records that Elijah:

> laid him on his own bed. Then he called out to the Lord. 'O Lord my God, is this thy care for the widow with whom I lodge, that thou hast been so cruel to her son? Then he breathed deeply upon the child three times and called on the Lord. 'O Lord my God, let the breath of life, I pray, return to the body of this child.' The Lord listened to Elijah's cry, and the breath of life returned to the child's body and he revived.

The account given of Elisha's healing is more detailed. It suggests that the boy may have been suffering from hypothermia and so needed warming up.

> Then getting on to the bed, he lay upon the child, put his mouth to the child's mouth, his eyes to his eyes and his hands to his hands: and, as he pressed upon him, the child's body grew warm. Elisha got up and walked once up and down the room; then getting on the bed again, he pressed upon him and breathed into him seven times; and the boy opened his eyes.

This early demonstration of mouth-to-mouth resuscitation anticipated, by over 2,000 years, best modern medical practice. It was only in the 1960s that positive pressure ventilation, by then a standard procedure in anaesthesia, became normal practice for dealing with emergencies such as cardiac arrest and drowning. We have no way of assessing what contribution the prophet's prayer made to the final outcome, but moments of crisis do call forth prayers for help and doctors are well aware of this, even though they prefer not to talk about it. In a published account of my own successful resuscitation of an old man in an isolated farmhouse, I was careful not to mention the intensity of the prayer I offered whilst travelling to the patient.[6]

Elisha and the Leper

Elisha had a special talent for healing. He restored the widow's son to life, provided an antidote for poisoned food[7] and cured Naaman of leprosy, though he did this almost contemptuously.[8] Naaman was a high-ranking Syrian general who was sent by his king to the King of Israel with a letter requesting him to heal Naaman of his disease. The king was afraid that the Syrians were trying to provoke a quarrel, but when Elisha heard the news he sent a message to the king saying that Naaman should be sent to him. When the Syrian general arrived at Elisha's house, the prophet sent his servant out to tell Naaman to wash seven times in the River Jordan. Naaman was furious. 'I thought,' he said 'that he would at least come out to me, pray to the Lord his God, wave his arm over the diseased spot, and cure me.' But his servants persuaded Naaman to accept the advice so he went and bathed in the river and was cured.

There are two points in this story that are of interest. First, spoken prayer, the laying on of hands and a contrite attitude were not necessary preliminaries for the healing. It occurred despite Naaman's anger and Elisha's insouciance. Second, the scientist in me cannot deny the possibility that Naaman did not have leprosy; he could have had a less serious affliction such as psoriasis, which would respond well to the sunlight while he bathed in the river. But whatever the nature of the disease or the treatment given, Elisha was a remarkable healer.

Jesus the Healer

Among the founders of the world religions, the status of Jesus is unique. A billion Christians worship him as Saviour and God Incarnate. Muslims revere him as a righteous prophet, and believe that he was miraculously born of Mary and that he ascended to heaven in bodily form. Members of the Baha'i Faith regard him as a 'Manifestation' of God, and those belonging to the Sufi branch of Islam refer to him as 'the wanderer and healer', an apt description for he travelled a great deal and healed many people.

Jesus' healing ministry was extremely well documented and must have made a powerful impact in the area at that time. The Gospels record thirty-five miraculous healings and about one-fifth of the text of the Gospels deals with this aspect of his ministry. There is no pattern to the healings; those who benefited included the blind, the deaf, the dumb, the lame and the paralytic. He also cured people suffering from leprosy, menorrhagia and epilepsy, and restored the dead to life. He was able to heal the sick both individually and as members of a group. Some of the reports mention that he touched the sick, or that he was touched by them, but physical contact does not seem to have been a necessary prerequisite. He was prepared to use physical aids as well, including clay mixed with his spittle which was a popular remedy for blindness at the time.[9] His healings were normally immediate and complete.

Botting suggests that 'most of the conditions that Jesus cured are still beyond the competence of medicine to cure'.[10] This is not true, though if he were alive today his healings might have a different range and pattern. Without diminishing the scope of his achievement, it is worth remembering that millions of people now have their sight restored by simple eye operations that were not available in biblical times, and that it has become routine practice to attempt the resuscitation of the clinically dead both inside and outside hospitals.

The Apostolic Era

There are many reports of miraculous healings in the early Christian Church. These are recorded mainly in the Gospels and Acts of the Apostles where, for instance, Luke writes:

> In the end the sick were actually carried out into the streets and laid there on beds and stretchers, so that even the shadow of Peter might fall on one or another as he passed by; and the people from the towns round Jerusalem flocked in bringing those who were ill or harassed by unclean spirits, and all of them were cured.[11]

Similarly of Paul, Luke wrote:

> Paul visited him and after prayer, laid his hands upon him and healed him: whereupon the other sick people on the island came also and were cured.[12]

In spite of these wonderful cures and marvellous healers, the early Christians still suffered from illnesses and did not expect all their diseases to be healed. The letters of the Apostles Paul, Peter, John and Jude to the early churches are full of instructions on how the members should behave but say little, or nothing, about physical healing: nor, with the exception of St James, do they offer any practical advice on the practice of healing. On the contrary, Paul writes that his companion Epaphroditus had been seriously ill and was to be sent home to Philippi,[13] and of another co-worker, Trophimus, that, 'I left Trophimus ill in Miletus'.[14]

Paul himself had a chronic ailment 'the thorn in his side', which he accepted as incurable, and advised his friend Timothy:

> Stop drinking nothing but water: take a little wine for your digestion, for your frequent ailments.[15]

St James had a more optimistic approach to intercessory prayer. In a letter he wrote:

Is one of you ill? he should send for the elders of the congregation to pray over him and anoint him with oil in the name of the Lord. The prayer offered in faith will save the sick man, the Lord will raise him from his bed, and any sins he may have committed will be forgiven. Therefore confess your sins to one another, and pray for one another, and then you will be healed.[16]

The Early Church

Early Christian literature is full of admonitions to care for the sick. Initially, this was accepted as a common burden, but by the third century, deacons and deaconesses had the specific duty of identifying those in need and reporting cases of sickness and poverty to the local bishop, and this remains one of their basic tasks. In the current service for the Ordination of Deacons, the Bishop tells candidates for the diaconate that 'A deacon is called to serve the Church of God, and to work with its members in caring for the poor, the needy, the sick, and all who are in trouble'[17]. The fourth century saw the building of the first Christian hospitals (*xenodochia*) one of the earliest and best known being the Basileias, which Basil the Great founded in Cappadocia in about 372. Of it, Gregory of Nazianus wrote:

behold the new city, the treasure house of godliness . . . in which disease is investigated and sympathy proved . . .We no longer have to look on the fearful and pitiable sight of men like corpses before death, with the greater parts of their limbs dead, driven from cities, from dwellings.[18]

Basil's hospital provided the model for many which were built throughout the eastern Roman Empire and then, in the fifth century, in Western Europe. The amenities included accommodation for travellers and a special section for lepers.

It has been suggested that the early Christians rejected medical treatment from secular practitioners, relying exclusively on the possibility of spiritual healing. It is probable that they used both approaches, accepting the help of physicians while at the same time continuing to seek, and claim, miraculous cures. The healing rites of the Early Church are similar to those used today, they are prayer, the laying-on of hands, baptism and the Eucharist. Of these, Caeserius of Arles (470–543) advised: 'Let him who is sick receive the body and blood of Christ and then let him anoint his body.' Basil the Great acknowledged the contribution that physical medicine could make to the health of his people when he wrote:

We must take great care to employ this medical art, if it should be necessary, not as making it wholly accountable for our state of health or illness, but as redounding to the greater glory of God . . .When reason allows we call in the doctor but we do not leave off hoping in God.

The same sentiment was evident when Origen (185–254) described medicine as 'beneficial and essential to mankind' and St John Chrysostom (354–407) referred to physicians as 'gifts of God'.[19]

Bede and the Celtic Church

We know that Celtic monks provided medicines for the sick and that clerics as well as laymen practised surgery, but miraculous healings also figured in contemporary records, most notably in those written by the first English historian, Bede (673–735). Rex Gardner, in his 1982 presidential address to the Newcastle and Northern Counties Medical Society, reviewed some of these healings, comparing them with modern 'miracle' cures. The seventh-century cases he cited included restoring the dead to life by prayer; healing intractable ulcers with holy salt, oil and prayer; and curing a nun, troubled by severe pains in the head, by anointing her with holy oil. In his consideration of these cures, Gardner accepted that there was no proof that any of these people had actually died before being revived or that they had been cured in the way mentioned, but he suggests that we should treat the accounts with greater respect than is the common practice. He made his point by setting alongside these ancient reports six contemporary claims of miraculous healings. One will be mentioned here.

A woman had a large varicose ulcer that had been troubling her for many years. The ulcer was getting worse and each morning her bandages were soaked in pus. Eventually, she asked for prayer at a monthly charismatic prayer meeting, where a doctor examined the leg and judged that, even if it were to heal, it would require skin grafting. At the meeting, two people prayed for her and by the next morning the ulcer had almost completely healed with normal skin covering, though one spot continued to exude pus. This area healed completely when a third person laid hands on the leg and prayed for her recovery. Most interestingly, the doctor who examined the leg at the prayer meeting was the President of the Society, Rex Gardner himself.[20]

Relics and Saints (Middle Ages)

There was a proliferation of miraculous cures in the early Middle Ages, often associated with shrines and the relics of saints. Within fifty years of his death, Bede himself was regarded as a saint and there were many claims that his relics had worked miraculous cures.[21] The literature of the Middle

Ages is full of such examples and 90 per cent of the miracles that were recorded at English shrines in the twelfth–fifteenth centuries involved healing or at least an improvement in the pilgrim's condition.[22]

Every shrine and monastery had its relics to which the faithful flocked, and these were often an important source of income to the monasteries and of healing to the visitors. The monastic cathedral dedicated to St Mary, St Osburg and All the Saints, which was founded at Coventry in 1043, and richly endowed by Lady Godiva and her husband Leofric, became famous for its beauty and the number of relics of the saints held there. These included the relics of St Osburg, which rested on a beam thickly coated with silver, and the arm of St Augustine of Hippo, which had been brought from Rome by the Archbishop of Canterbury and presented by him to Earl Leofric. The inventory included:

- A part of the Holy Cross, in silver and gilt.
- Our Lady's milk, in a silver and gilt container.
- A piece of Our Lady's tomb.
- St Osborne's head enclosed in copper and gilt.
- A silver cross set in stones with a relic of St James.
- An arm of St Justyn, in silver.
- A rib of St Laurence, in silver.
- A barrel of relics of confessors, of copper.
- A large necklace of precious stones, donated by Lady Godiva: this was hung on the image of St Mary, 'so that those that come of Devotion thither should say as many prayers as were gems therein'.[23]

In 1539, this centre of pilgrimage was closed by Henry VIII, its treasures were absorbed into his treasury and its walls subsequently used as a quarry for new building projects.

It is impossible today to appreciate the importance of such shrines in the Middle Ages, but there is no doubt that they played a significant role in the healing culture of that period. Moreover the use, for healing purposes, of objects associated with the saints has some biblical authority for in the Acts of the Apostles, we learn:

> And through Paul God worked singular miracles: when handkerchiefs and scarves which had been in contact with his skin were carried to the sick, they were rid of their diseases and the evil spirits came out of them.[24]

Such ideas were vigorously denounced in the Reformation by Protestant divines, so it is interesting to note that the practice was revived in the twentieth century, by charismatic evangelists such as Oral Roberts.

The Reformation (Sixteenth Century)

Amundsen, in his account of the religious scene in the early Middle Ages (500–1050) tells us: 'The cult of saints and relics was the single most important force in the conversion of Western Europe.'[25] This assessment by a leading historian may be controversial, but the situation had certainly changed by the seventeenth century. Various factors were at work to make changes inevitable. Most notable was the Black Death (1348–49), the most dreadful pestilence ever to afflict Europe: it ravaged the populations in town and countryside alike, killing at least a third of those living at the time, and especially enclosed institutions such as the monasteries which, now emptied of monks, were never able to re-establish their former position in society. Within Christianity itself, important doctrinal splits became evident and there were increasing demands for the Church to reform itself.

An important catalyst in this period of change was the publication of the Gutenburg Bible in 1455. Now books were no longer the preserve of a few learned monks. They became available to a much wider reading public and a new attitude to the Scriptures developed within the Protestant branch of the Church, with the written Word of God replacing the sacraments and priesthood as the supreme and ultimate authority in the Church.

The Protestants adopted the viewpoint that the age of miracles had passed, that healing miracles were a particular feature of the Early Church and that whilst God was the Great Physician who shared our sufferings with us, He had also given us physicians and physic to counter the illnesses, diseases and pestilence prevalent in the earthly sphere. They taught that the healing miracles recorded in the Bible were not random events; they happened at strategic and unique stages in the unfolding of God's redemptive purpose, and that the key stages in the Old Testament were:

1. The Exodus.
2. The ministries of Elijah and Elisha.
3. The Babylonian exile in particular the experiences of Daniel and his companions.

The key stages in the New Testament were:

1. The earthly ministry of Christ.
2. The proclamation of the Gospel message by the Apostles.

These ideas, developed by Protestants during the Reformation, are still held by Evangelical Churches today. They came to believe that the unique range of healing miracles recorded in the New Testament were designed specifically to authenticate Jesus of Nazareth as the Christ, the Son of God and Redeemer of the world. The later miracles found in the Acts of the

Apostles, underlined the credentials of the Apostles as witnesses of Christ as they established His Church and spread the Gospel message to a pagan world. The purpose of the miracles was to attest to key stages in salvation history.

It is worth emphasizing that evangelical Christians continue to affirm that miracles are rare today, a view that was held by mainstream Protestant Churches until quite recently. While not denying that God can still work miracles, the underlying principle remains unchanged, and in writing on this subject in the *Evangelical Times* Eryl Davies affirmed 'that it is extremely difficult to find any convincing evidence that modern, so-called miracles of healing are genuine'.[26] He also makes two other pertinent observations. First, that the Bible warns us that faith should not be based on a healing or a miracle but on the Word of God; second, to remember that healing is not necessarily the work of God, as there is good biblical evidence that the devil and his hosts are also capable of 'signs' and healing miracles.

I find his second point quite unacceptable and if his suggestion that there could be a connection between healing and the devil were taken seriously, then the consequences for hospitals and health centres would be considerable as they would have to take steps to counteract the risk of any such malign influence. This would be reminiscent of the attitude that fuelled the witch-hunts of the Middle Ages, though the roots of that terror can be traced back to an earlier period.

Healing and Witchcraft

Once Christianity became a state religion under Constantine in 313, various councils, starting with the Synod of Ancyra in 314, issued decrees forbidding the practice of healing outside the jurisdiction of the Church. The purpose was to outlaw pagan practices, but it was not always clear what was un-Christian and therefore illicit. Augustine of Hippo (354–430), for instance, considered it permissible to eat herbs for stomach pains but not to wear herbs around the neck for the same purpose: the latter was a superstitious charm. However, the full authority of the Church and State was not directed against such magical practices until much later. Inexorably, beginning with the first medical licentiates in the twelfth and thirteenth centuries and the subsequent development of medical and surgical guilds, the practice of medicine ceased to be a universal right and became a privilege that excluded unlicensed practitioners. Those who continued in their unsanctioned attempts to bring relief to the sick were increasingly regarded as witches.

Before the Reformation, two types of witchcraft were recognized in medieval Europe: white witchcraft, which included the practice of healing, and *maleficium* – black magic. *Maleficium* included sorcery – the manipulation of objects by the power of thought and the incantation of words – and also the invocation of powers, activated by hatred, to cause harm to other people. After the fifteenth century a third type of witch became identified, one who had made a pact with and sold her soul to the devil. The use of the female gender is particularly appropriate here as most of the people condemned as witches were women. In contrast, the witch hunters, court officials and executioners were all men.

With the Reformation there came a hardening of attitude towards the healing practised by ordinary people and traditional healers, an increase in hostility that was most noticeable in Protestant countries. In Catholic countries shrines associated with healings continued to be a focus of religious devotion, but in Protestant countries their desecration had left a void that was filled by a variety of practices that became increasingly labelled as of the devil, or witchcraft.[27] During the sixteenth and seventeenth centuries, there was an upsurge in witch trials amounting almost to epidemic proportions. The most severe persecutions were in Germany and France, but notable witch-hunts occurred in America, Ireland, Scandinavia and Scotland. Such hunts were relatively minor affairs in England, whilst Spain, with the exception of the Basque country, and southern Italy avoided them almost completely, possibly because of the continued reverence the Catholic Church accorded its saints and their shrines.

The English Parliament passed its first repressive Act against witchcraft only in 1542. As a direct result of this Act English witches were persecuted in large numbers but, because English law was different from and not subject to the relentless rigour of Scottish and Continental (European) law, English witches were rarely tortured to extract confessions. English lawyers continued to maintain the distinction between white and black magic, and this was reflected in the severity of the punishment meted out. The demonic pact was seldom mentioned.

The revised Witchcraft Act of 1563, passed in the reign of Elizabeth Tudor, imposed the death penalty on those found guilty of merely consulting a witch whilst a new Act in 1642 was even more severe and would have increased the risk for healers and those seeking help from them. The British Parliament repealed these and all other Acts against sorcery in 1735, but the Witchcraft Act of 1735 still made it illegal to act as a spiritual medium, practise clairvoyance, telepathy or any similar power, including spiritual healing. This Act was repealed only in 1951 when it was replaced by the Fraudulent Medium Act, which permitted the above practices but only if they were not undertaken for any reward or were practised solely for the purpose of entertainment. It was only then that attendance at a Spiritualist Church and its healing services ceased to be illegal in the United Kingdom.

The Blesser and the King

It was a terrifying experience to be arraigned as a witch. Self-styled witch-finders received payment for each conviction and they used a variety of methods to identify their victims. These included pricking their flesh with needles to find numb areas, searching for the Devil's mark on their bodies and accepting any malicious gossip about them. There was also the ordeal by water: if the submerged victim drowned she was not a witch but if she survived the ducking, she was.

Henry Baggillie was an unlicensed healer or 'blesser' who was brought before the magistrates in Lancashire in May 1664 on a charge of witchcraft. He had been taught by his father certain words and prayers which, if repeated, would help any sick person or animal in their extremity. The words were:

> I tell thee forespoken toothe and tonge,
> hearte and hearte ralthe,
> three things thee boote moste,
> the father sonne and holighuoste.

After this recitation he said the Lord's Prayer and the Creed three times. Baggillie had used these words to bless his friends and their cattle. He claimed that all those he had blessed had recovered and that he had received no payment other than a bit of bread and cheese or similar 'commodity'. The magistrate's note on the recording document says simply 'Witchcrafte'.[28]

In contrast the ruling sovereign was permitted, even expected, to heal. The Royal Touch for the King's Evil dates back to St Louis IX of France and Edward III of England, possibly even to Edward the Confessor. It was regarded as a cure for epilepsy and scrofula, a tuberculous disease of the neck glands. The Stuart kings were happy to continue with the custom as it re-enforced the idea of the Divine Right of Kings, and although Charles I was beheaded, people still believed monarchs possessed the power to heal. His son, Charles II, is said to have touched almost 100,000 people during his reign and the practice continued into the reign of Queen Anne (1702–14), who touched the infant Dr Samuel Johnson, but was eventually stopped by her Hanoverian successors.

There is no evidence that the Royal Touch cured anyone, but people probably felt better for being in close contact with their sovereign just as now an audience with the Pope, or meeting the Queen or Nelson Mandela, can be an uplifting experience. There is one important difference however. The Royal Touch was associated with a special religious office, 'At the Healing', and this remained an integral part of the Book of Common Prayer until the eighteenth century.[29]

George Fox (Seventeenth Century)

The seventeenth century was a very turbulent period in European history and witches were not the only victims of reforming zeal. In Britain family loyalties were sharply divided by the conflict between King and Parliament, and by disputes between the Churches. Being a Catholic priest was a capital offence and Philip Evans, John Lloyd and David Lewis were just three of the priests who were hanged, drawn and quartered in the 1670s. Yet the same century saw important developments in science and literature, Sir Isaac Newton formulated the law of gravity, William Harvey showed how the blood circulated around the body, Shakespeare wrote his plays and John Milton wrote *Paradise Lost*. During the English civil war, John Milton supported the parliamentary cause but his contemporary, George Fox, the founder of the Religious Society of Friends (Quakers), was of a different persuasion.

George Fox (1624–91) was an outstanding religious leader and a remarkable healer. The son of a weaver, he became a shoemaker and then dedicated most of his life to preaching. He was firmly opposed to war, to formality in religious observance and to the taking of oaths. He was often imprisoned for his outspoken opinions. Fox was a gentle person of great courage, who visited and supported slaves in the West Indies and the North American Indians, pointing out that they shared with him and the rest of humanity an inner spark of Divine Light. This was at a time when it was not unusual for men to say that women had no souls.

He travelled widely in Europe too and is often likened to St Paul, as their experiences as preachers, prisoners and healers seem so similar.[30] Both men were prolific writers and Fox's Journal and letters are still studied by scholars interested in the English social history of the seventeenth century.

Our primary interest is with Fox the healer, an aspect of his life which has been well documented most recently in a booklet by Hodges, which mentions the healing of Margaret Rouse's child. Fox was Margaret Rouse's stepfather and when her daughter became critically ill with smallpox he went to visit the child. As he stood by the bedside he felt the presence of the Lord's power and went away content but visited again the next day at the mother's request. Of this he wrote:

> I saw the child was full of the power of the Lord and it rested upon it and rested in it. And at night it died. And after the spirit of the child had appeared to me and there was a mighty substance of a glorious life in that child and I bid her mother be content, for it was well, and it was well that she had such an innocent offering for the Lord. And she was finely settled and contented through the will of the Lord.[31]

Most people would not regard this as a healing, but from Fox's perspective it was, as he was able to reassure the mother of the child's spiritual well-being. We do not know whether this helped her to come to terms with her loss, but there is evidence that those who profess a strong spiritual belief resolve their grief more rapidly and completely following bereavement than other people.[32]

Fox's friend John Banks has also provided a detailed account of Fox's healing power. He describes in his journal how he experienced pain of such severity in his shoulder and arm that he was unable to dress himself. This persisted for three months and during this time the arm and hand began to wither. He could obtain no relief from the doctors, so he went to Fox, and after attending a Quaker meeting they walked together for a short distance. Then Fox placed his hand on Banks's shoulder and prayed: 'The Lord strengthen thee both within and without.' Then they parted and Banks went to a friend's house for the night. During supper he found that he could use his hand and that the pain had gone. The next day he returned home 'with my hand and arm restored to former use and strength without any pain'.[33] When he told Fox at their next meeting his friend said, 'Well John, give God the glory.'

Fox also healed his own mother of the 'palsy' so that she regained her strength on the side of the body that had been weakened by a stroke and was immediately able to resume her normal activities.

Fox was a prolific writer and his Journals were published within three years of his death by Milton's secretary. This contrasts markedly with the decision taken at the same time not to publish his *Book of Miracles*, which contained his account of about 150 miraculous healings. It took nearly 200 years for its contents to come into the public domain and people do wonder why the book was suppressed. I offer two possible explanations. First, that scepticism was so rife that his executors doubted whether readers would accept that such healings could take place; the other thought takes into account the politico-religious and social climate of that period. A very repressive Witchcraft Act had been passed in 1642 and these were dangerous times for Dissenters and anyone holding unusual political or religious views. There was a very real risk of being brought before magistrates and imprisoned. It was not always easy to draw the line between healing and witchcraft and the Society of Friends would not wish to be linked with the latter. The publication of the *Book of Miracles* might have produced a response that the leaders of the Society of Friends considered undesirable and for that reason they chose not to publish it. It was about this time also that the Royal Touch was discontinued and it is worth noting that John Wesley, the most influential religious leader of the eighteenth century and a man who was very interested in all matters medical, made no claim to be a healer.

Chapter Five
Healing: The Field Widens

It is difficult for us to appreciate just how limited scientific knowledge was in the eighteenth century. A physician's knowledge of anatomy would have been at best rudimentary and people still thought in terms of four basic elements – earth, air, fire and water. Nothing was known about the chemical elements, but interest in scientific research was increasing and hydrogen was recognized as a distinct substance in 1766 and nitrogen in 1772. Shortly afterwards, Joseph Priestley demonstrated the existence of oxygen, but scientists were still unaware that this newly discovered gas was essential for life.

This was a time when healers were to be found in a wide range of occupations and professions, and the mentally disturbed were likely to be treated by clergymen or astrologers, physicians or magicians. Treatment might involve religious counsel and exorcism, drugs and prayer, therapeutic regimes and the provision of amulets and charms to protect against demonic influences.[1] The clergy were expected to minister to the sick and it was not unusual for a clergyman to have trained as a doctor, a tradition exemplified by Thomas Secker who became Archbishop of Canterbury having taken his medical degree at Leyden in 1721.

But training in medicine was becoming more arduous as it became more scientific, and increasingly the practice of the healing arts was to become a speciality in itself. At the same time, society was undergoing a massive reorganization: the last quarter of the century was to see the emergence of a United States of America and of a Republic in France. Less dramatically, the scene was set for the introduction of smallpox vaccination and the practice of homeopathy as well as the advent of many new religious sects, which would later have a decisive effect on attitudes to healing.

Methodism (Eighteenth Century)

Methodism can trace its origins back to the Oxford of the 1720s when John and Charles Wesley joined a group of like-minded students intent on recapturing the spirit of the early Christian Church. It did not make much of an impact until 1738 when its founder, John Wesley (1703–91), returned to England from America, where he had been suspended from his chaplaincy in Georgia following a scandalous love affair. Shortly after his return, he attended a Moravian church in London where he underwent a conversion experience and began to create local Methodist societies. These mushroomed in number and size so that the total membership had reached 100,000 when he died in 1791. By this time, parallel American societies had established themselves as an independent Church and the English Methodists did the same the following year.

John Wesley was fascinated by medical matters and was probably more closely involved in the practice of medicine than any other major figure in Christendom. He was reading medical textbooks at the age of seventeen whilst a student at Oxford, and studied medicine seriously for several months in 1731 before he went, as a missionary, to the New World. He published many tracts on medical subjects, including *Thoughts on the Sin of Onan* (masturbation); *A Dissertation on the Gout* and *Thoughts on Nervous Disorders*. His best known work was *Primitive Physick*, which was published in 1747. This became so popular that twenty-four editions of the book had been printed in America and eighty-eight in England by 1880.

The advice he gave in *Primitive Physick* was based on common sense and much of what he said about diet, cleanliness and exercise is to be found in the articles written today by dietitians and journalists. He also had some views peculiar to his period. Among the remedies he advocated were cold baths, toad pills and warm puppies on the belly. He was interested in the possibility that the judicious use of electricity could have a role in healing and opened clinics where 'electrical therapy' was one of the treatments. He recommended occasional fasting and the avoidance of rich foods, but he did not condemn the consumption of moderate amounts of wine and beer – that proscription came later in the history of Methodism – but he condemned spirits as 'a certain though slow poison'.

Wesley regarded the care of the sick as an indispensable part of Methodism and an activity particularly suited to women. He opened dispensaries for poor people and practised medicine himself, a custom that Methodist ministers followed well into the nineteenth century. Wesley had no compunction about prescribing drugs and often did so, but for him the most effective drug was prayer. In his letters he refers to miraculous cures and these included people suffering from leprosy, paralysis and infectious diseases. He was deeply interested in people's physical welfare but he always claimed that the greatest miracles he saw were the wholly trans-formed lives of people led to love and trust God completely.[2]

A brief review of Methodism naturally tends to focus on John Wesley but the hymns written by his brother Charles (1707–88) are of great therapeutic value and this needs to be emphasized. Music, especially singing in unison, gives solace to the grieving heart and it is impossible to measure the comfort that Charles' hymns have brought to people who were dispirited, depressed and filled with a sense of hopelessness. As his contemporary, William Congreve wrote:[3] 'Music hath charms to soothe a savage breast, / To soften rocks, or bend a knotted oak'. However, whilst the healing power of music has always been recognized, it is rarely given a significant place in the physician's armamentarium. In modern times, the practice of music therapy is mainly to be found in mental hospitals, but there are signs that the value of this approach is also welcomed in hospices, a development that is largely due to the initiative of the artists who offer their services freely in palliative care centres and to the work done by the Council for Music in Hospitals.

Music also has a contribution to make in geriatric care. Wardle says that singing well-known hymns or songs can help people, when their speech has been impaired by a stroke, to regain some facility with words and sounds. He considers the 'semi-supine' position to be the ideal one for listening to music or for meditation, and describes a combination of music (preferably Mozart) and the adoption of a semi-supine position as almost 'heaven on earth'.[4]

Homeopathy

There is something essentially English about the Methodist Church but it is difficult to say the same about homeopathy. We tend to be insular and this has a wider, more continental appeal. Like Methodism, homeopathic medicine appeared before scientific medicine had taken its first stumbling steps and even before Laennec (1781–1826) had invented the stethoscope. It was the brainchild of Samuel Hahnemann, a German physician who was working in Leipzig in 1790 when he noted that the symptoms presented by patients suffering from malaria were similar to the effects produced in a healthy person if they were given quinine, then the treatment of choice for malaria. This observation gave him the idea that 'like cures like'; in other words, that diseases are best treated by agents that produce symptoms of the disease in a healthy person. So a person suffering from hay fever may be prescribed *Allium cepa*, a derivative of the common onion, because onions produce the irritation and watering of the eyes and the clear nasal discharge that occur in hay fever.

Hahnemann was convinced that drugs were more effective if taken in minute quantities. Accordingly, homeopathists prescribe minuscule doses of the active agent for their patients. They achieve this by serial dilution of the medicine and by succussion, vigorous shaking, which they believe increases the potency of the drug. As a consequence, many homeopathic medicines are ultramolecular;[5] in other words, they are diluted to such an extent that not a single molecule of the prescribed drug is likely to be present in the final product offered to the patient. Hahnemann also taught that the patient and not the disease should be the focus of attention. as a 'vital principle' animates and pervades the body and disease occurs if its flow is disrupted.

Homeopathy was very popular in the nineteenth century and is experiencing a minor renaissance today. About 1,000 doctors and 1,500 practitioners, who have no conventional healthcare background, practise this branch of medicine in the United Kingdom. It is also very popular in mainland Europe where about 10,000 German and French doctors offer this approach to their patients. They are likely to take a detailed history of the patient's complaint and may ask if the symptoms vary with factors such as the weather, diet, mood or time of day. The intention is to form a 'symptom picture' which will enable the physician to prescribe a suitable remedy from the homeopathic *Materia medica*. Some homeopathists use dowsing as an aid to diagnosis and treatment. They do this by holding a short pendulum over the patient, or the possible remedy, and then reach a decision by observing its swing.

The Early Mormons (Nineteenth Century)

The beginning of the nineteenth century saw the emergence of a surprisingly large number of religious movements, most notably in North America and Japan. The founder was usually a lay person who experienced a mystical experience of such grandeur that they felt impelled to preach this new truth and almost coincidentally attracted disciples. This seems to have been the case when Joseph Smith (1805–44), a twenty-five-year-old farmer, established The Church of Jesus Christ of Latter-Day Saints (The Mormons) in upstate New York, in 1830.

Smith's mystical experiences began in 1820 when he had a vision of God the Father and of Jesus Christ as two separate beings. He was later to have encounters with the Angel Moroni (in 1823) and John the Baptist (in 1829) and to receive the *Book of Mormon* which believers consider as much the word of God as the Bible. He was assassinated in 1844 having led his followers on a prolonged journey into a remote area of Illinois. Some of his

followers settled there, but many decided to continue westward and undertook the great trek to Utah under the leadership of Brigham Young
(1801–77).

These early pioneers had many difficulties to overcome, including a
whole range of diseases and injuries not normally encountered in present-
day western societies, and they had few doctors to provide the medical
skills needed. Consequently when members of the Church fell ill, Smith
and his followers turned for guidance to the Bible and, in particular, to the
advice of St James:

> If there are any sick among you, Let him call for the elders of the church: and
> let them pray over him, anointing him with oil in the name of the Lord: and
> the prayer of faith shall save the sick, and the Lord shall raise him up.

This advice was supported by further revelations, which specifically
commanded the church elders to exercise this gift of healing, and another,
which stated:

> whoso shall ask it in my name, in faith, they shall cast out devils; they shall
> heal the sick; they shall cause the blind to receive their sight and the deaf to
> hear, and the dumb to speak, and the lame to walk.[6]

People went to the elders for healing, and healing ordinances are still an
important and regular feature of life within the Mormon community,
though not in a public setting.

Consecrated oil is used for the healing rite, which nowadays is normally
performed in the patient's home though it may be undertaken in other
places such as a church, hospital or nursing home. Two priests of the
Order of Melchizedek are always present, one to anoint while the other
acts as a witness. This requirement is not as exclusive as it might seem,
since most adult male members of the Church belong to this order of
priesthood. There are two distinct parts to the service. First, the anointing
with oil, when one of the priests, usually a close relative, places oil on the
crown of the patient's head. This is followed by the sealing when both men
'lay their hands on the individual's head' and bless and pray for him/her in
the name of Jesus.

The demand for healing was so high in the early days that one prominent member, Wilford Woodruff, recorded over 1,000 instances in which
he was personally involved. He wrote:

> Many were healed by the power of God. Devils were cast out, the dumb
> spake, the deaf heard, the blind saw, the lame walked, the sick were raised up
> and in one instance the dead were raised in the Case of my own wife After
> the spirit left her body.[7]

The casting out of devils seems to have been an almost commonplace event at that time and the first miraculous cure recorded by the Church took place when Joseph Smith held the hand of a convert who was convulsing and 'rebuked the devil'. The victim immediately spoke out and said that he could see the devil leave him and vanish from his sight. An unusual practice in the early Church was the use of rebaptism as an aid to healing. There was no clear precedent for this and it was soon discarded. However, I have watched an open-air service in which members of an American Baptist Church chose to be rebaptized even though they were not sick. A similar urge to recommitment is apparent when ministers of religion renew their ordination vows or married couples their marriage vows though I find the motives for doing so obscure once such a vow has been solemnly given.

Women are not allowed to perform the ordinances prescribed for elders in the Church of Jesus Christ of Latter-Day Saints, but it seems likely that during the pioneering days some did practise healing and, according to Wilford Woodruff, often with 'miraculous results'.[8] To some extent the practice continues as the 'laying-on of hands' by women is accepted as a form of healing, though they may not anoint, nor do they 'seal' in the way that priesthood bearers do. There is some evidence that members of the early Church spoke in tongues and, from a medical viewpoint, I would regard this as helpful and cathartic and an aid to good health. Speaking in tongues still occurs within the Church but it always has to be interpreted, otherwise it is regarded as of no value and just gibberish. I am uncertain about this as I remember a Presbyterian minister telling me many years ago that he had the gift of tongues but only practised it in private, usually in the car, as it might otherwise upset his congregation. He said it was a most helpful gift, which enabled him to continue his work in the Church with greater joy and effectiveness.

Like John Wesley, the early Mormons tended to be antipathetic towards orthodox medical practice but this attitude was changing by the 1870s when, at the behest of Brigham Young, young members were sent for training to the medical schools in the Eastern states. There have been many other changes in the community, including the abandonment of polygamy in 1890. Mormons have a reputation for 'working hard and playing hard' and the effectiveness of their lifestyle in reducing the incidence of cancer, heart disease and several other disorders is well documented. Much of this can be credited to the proscription of tobacco and alcohol – particularly the former – and healthy diets, as well as lower levels of promiscuity and early childbearing. There is also a network of professional psychologists and counsellors who are available to help church leaders deal with any emotional problems that may trouble the membership.

Christian Science

People became Mormons because they were caught by the vision of Joseph Smith, not because they wanted to be healthy, but it was the evidence of physical healing – of the deaf hearing, the blind regaining their sight, the lame walking and cancerous growths being resolved – that first attracted people to Christian Science.[9] Other religious denominations have claimed similar successes, but the philosophy underlying the Christian Science approach to healing is quite different from that of most Churches where the emphasis is on prayer, the laying on of hands and healing by grace. In Christian Science, healing is achieved not by asking God to cure someone of an illness but by believing that the illness does not exist. The teaching is that people only think that they have cancer or migraine or bronchitis. These are delusions, imaginary concepts lacking reality, which disappear when confronted with correct understanding and clear thinking. A similar approach is adopted to those malign influences that cause distress by disrupting a person's family, social or professional life, for instance bereavement or redundancy.

Christian Science has always had an intense interest in health and how it is best maintained. Its members have stressed the importance of healing as part of the Church's ministry more than any other religious group and its founder anticipated the present interest in spiritual healing well before the Pentecostal movement popularized the practice. Yet the significant role that Christian Science has played in this development has been largely, and often deliberately, ignored by other Churches.

Christian Science emerged after the American Civil War (1861–65) and was a direct result of the experiences of its founder, Mary Baker Eddy (1821–1910). She has been aptly described as a 'wounded healer who has been there and knows the way out'.[10] Born in New Hampshire, she grew up in a strict Calvinistic household but was never able to accept its doctrines on hell and predestination. A sickly child, she had little formal education but was writing both prose and poetry at an early age. She married three times. Her first husband died of yellow fever, her second was a philanderer whom she divorced, and she finally married Asa Eddy, a sewing-machine salesman. He gave her a great deal of support and helped her with the promotion of her new religion, but it was her second husband, Daniel Patterson, who sowed the seeds of the movement by introducing her to Phineas Quimby, a clockmaker and hypnotist, who cured her of a crippling disease in 1863. Quimby was among the foremost hypnotists of his day and worked on the principle that the underlying cause of all disease was the faulty mental attitude of the sufferer. He attributed his healing skills to clear thinking and the ability to gain a patient's confidence in his capacity to heal. These were ideas that interested Mary Baker Patterson even though she did not entirely agree with them.

Quimby died in 1866. About a month later Mary Baker slipped on the ice and was so badly hurt that she felt unable to leave her bed. The exact nature of her injuries is not known but the homeopathic doctor she consulted could do nothing to relieve her distress, ascribing the problem to internal injuries. In desperation, she turned to the Bible for help. She was reading the Gospels, and the healing miracles performed by Jesus, when she had a wonderful revelation. It was as if 'a flood of light poured into her' and she was suddenly aware 'of the spiritual perfection of the universe as it exists in the mind of God'.[11] She realized that she had been given a new view of reality, similar to the truth preached and practised by Jesus, 'that there is but one creation, which is wholly spiritual'. This is the basic tenet that distinguishes the Christian Science approach to healing from that of other healing groups.

The effect on her illness was instantaneous. She immediately got out of bed, completely healed. Her friends regarded her cure as miraculous, but she looked upon it as a manifestation of a divine law. The next few years were difficult. She was separated from her second husband, had no permanent home and no regular income, but she had a few followers who later became successful healers. She spent much of this period reading the Bible, refining her healing techniques and consolidating the ideas about reality, divine law, sin and sickness which, she believed, God had revealed to her. She also lectured, saw patients and wrote various pamphlets on healing.

In 1875, she published *Science and Health*, the textbook of Christian Science, which she later revised and reissued as *Science and Health with Key to the Scriptures*. In 1891, she founded the Massachusetts Metaphysical College where she taught until it was closed in 1899. By this time she had already established the First Church of Christ, Scientist in Boston and branch churches were soon flourishing in other cities. Central to her philosophy and teaching was the idea that only God exists. Nothing exists apart from Him. The universe and all its contents, including men and women, are just perfect ideas proceeding from God and reflections of His harmonious and eternal nature. God alone exists and He is Spirit, perfect in love and goodness. Matter does not exist; therefore evil, disease and death are concepts that are not based on reality.[12]

The basic beliefs of Christian Science were set out in the 1880s and have undergone little change since then. They encapsulate most of Christian teaching including acceptance of:

- the Bible as 'our sufficient guide to eternal life;
- the Doctrine of the Trinity;
- the forgiveness of sins;

- Jesus' atonement as the evidence of divine efficacious Love;
- the fact that man is saved through Christ, through Truth, Life and Love as demonstrated by Jesus in healing the sick, and overcoming sin and death.[13]

But crucially, however, they reject the reality of matter and evil.

Christian Science should, in theory, be able to deal with all manner of complaints but whilst members make little use of medical services they are free to do so. Most are willing to wear spectacles, receive dental and obstetric care and accept conventional treatment for major injuries. They run their own sanatoriums for rest and nursing care, and pursue a generally healthy life-style eating moderately well and avoiding habit-forming drugs including alcohol, cannabis and tobacco.

Christian Scientists who feel ill are able to seek help from a 'practitioner', who will discuss the situation and pray with them. Practitioners are church members who have received a short, though intensive, course of training to prepare them for this specialized role. They will also have attended the two weeks of 'class instruction' that is normally undertaken by Christian Scientists at some stage, and they will continue to immerse themselves in the Bible and the writings of Christian Science, especially *Science and Health with Key to the Scriptures*. The main purpose of this course is to instil the habit of study and prayer which will enable students to pursue the lifelong discipline of spiritual growth essential for serious seekers. Although the 'practitioner's' course is short, graduates receive a Bachelor of Christian Science degree and may use the letters CSB after their names.[14]

Christian Science services are very simple and low-key. They are usually held on Sundays and on one evening during the week. There is no sermon, this being replaced by readings from the Bible and from *Science and Health with Key to the Scriptures*. An important function of the weekday service is to enable church members to testify in public to the healing that they have received. This is always done in a very quiet, matter-of-fact manner. The Christian Science press publishes thousands of testimonials to the efficacy of Christian Science healing. These tend to follow a pattern: beginning with a brief résumé of the individual's association with Christian Science, followed by a description of the illness and cure, and finally an expression of gratitude to Christian Science for the blessings received.

Typical concluding remarks are as follows:

> I've led a very vigorous life since that time and have continued to turn to God as my only physician.

> The healing has been permanent and I have had complete freedom of movement in all of my many activities.

I have continued to rely on prayer in Christian Science for healing in all the years since.

With joy I noticed that after I had begun regular study of the Bible Lesson in *Christian Science Quarterly*, my general state of health took a substantial turn for the better.[15]

Osteopathy and Chiropractic

The end of the nineteenth century saw many new developments in the field of patient care, some of which were incorporated into mainstream medical practice. This was the period when Sigmund Freud and Carl Jung were taking their first, tentative steps into the deeper regions of the human psyche. In so doing, they were laying the foundations of our present system of psychotherapy and, more recently, of the extensive networks of volunteer helpers trained to listen to the problems of the distressed.

Other innovators were turning their attention to the basic framework of the human body. It is worth emphasizing, before going into the details of these specialities, that treatment by the manipulation of bones had been practised in the United States and Britain long before the advent of osteopathy. Its practitioners were the spiritual heirs of the bonesetters who for hundreds of years had plied their trade across Europe, and their skill and dedication provided a rich legacy for the twentieth century. Some of their techniques have become part of medical practice.

Hugh Owen Thomas (1834–91), the man generally recognized as the Father of Orthopaedic Surgery, was a Liverpool surgeon who came from a long line of bonesetters based in Anglesey, North Wales.

Sir Herbert Barker (1869–1950) was another famous practitioner with the 'magic touch'. He was not a medical man but learned the art of bone-setting while apprenticed to his cousin, John Atkinson, one of the foremost practitioners of his day. Atkinson's patients included celebrities such as the Polish pianist and composer Ignace Paderewski. Barker inherited Atkinson's practice in 1905. He established his clinic in central London and was so successful that he attracted an impressive clientele, including members of Royalty, Dukes, artists like Augustus John, Indian princes, leading sportsmen and even Princess Marie Louise's cat whose dislocated jaw he reduced. He was knighted in 1922 after the Prime Minister had received letters recommending such an action from many senior doctors, including a former president of the Royal College of Surgeons and Sir Alfred Fripp, surgeon-in-ordinary to the King.[16]

It was possibly the American Civil War that was the spur for the concepts behind osteopathy and chiropractic gaining a higher profile in the United States. Andrew Taylor Still (1828–1917), the founder of osteopathy, was a physician who had served with the Confederate forces. The distress he experienced during that time was to be compounded later when three of his children died in an epidemic. He must have felt that his medical training was, in some way, inadequate because, in 1874, the year before Mary Baker Eddy wrote *Science and Health*, he published the principles of osteopathy. He had hoped that his thesis would be acceptable to the medical establishment but none of the medical schools could find room for his ideas in their curriculum and so, in 1882, he opened his own school in Kirksville, Missouri and conferred the degree of Doctor of Osteopathy (DO) on its graduates. The professional training it provides is now similar to that of doctors and, in the United States, osteopathic physicians are licensed to practise medicine in all the States, usually with the same professional rights and responsibilities as holders of the MD degree.

The founders of osteopathy and chiropractic both believed, like Samuel Hahnemann, that a 'vital force' permeates and animates the body and that disease is the result of a disturbance in its flow. They also emphasized the importance of correcting disorders in the musculo-skeletal system, particularly the spine, as an essential step in restoring health. Chiropractic was the brainchild of an American merchant, D. D. Palmer. He had originally been a 'magnetic healer' who had achieved a notable success when he cured a man of deafness by realigning his cervical vertebrae. He went on to establish his own system of therapeutics before he died in 1913, and chiropractic is now a highly respected profession and practitioners are found in many countries throughout the world.

It is sometimes said that osteopathy is a gentler technique than chiropractic and I think this is probably true. The main difference is that the traditional chiropractor uses a short, sharp thrust to the joint when manipulating the spine, whilst osteopaths prefer to apply force in a less direct way, using a 'long-lever' approach. An increasing number of chiropractors are now using the McTimoney Technique, which was devised by an English practitioner, John McTimoney, who opened his own chiropractic school in Oxfordshire, in 1972. It has a four-year course, which is validated by the University of Wales. One of its most interesting features is its postgraduate course in animal manipulation. This two-year course was launched in 1998 in consultation with the Royal College of Veterinary Surgeons.

The McTimoney technique is considered to be a return to 'pure chiropractic'. It emphasizes the importance of sensitive hands and 'touch' in diagnosis rather than the use of X-rays, which has become almost a routine procedure for many chiropractors. Stress is also placed on speed, dexterity and accuracy when readjusting the bones.

Its main method of manipulation is called the toggle–torque–recoil. The toggle is the thrust, the torque is the twisting movement applied with the thrust, and the recoil is the quick removal of the hands from the patient's body. Andrews and Courtenay say that the 'depth at which practitioners are taught sensitivity of touch and palpation skills probably exceeds that of other manipulative techniques'.[17] I do not know if this claim can be validated, but they also say that McTimoney practitioners are likely to have 'a spiritual or at least strongly intuitive', approach, and that I find interesting.

Pentecostal Healing

The turn of the century was a time of ferment and not only in medical circles. It also witnessed the beginnings of the Pentecostal movement, one of the most conspicuous religious developments of the twentieth century. No one can say precisely where it started, but most likely it flowed from the Azusa Street Mission in Los Angeles where, in 1906, the black holiness preacher William J. Seymour ignited a revival of astonishing intensity, in which people of many races and backgrounds testified to the glory of Jesus Christ and manifested the spiritual gifts of tongues, healings and prophecies. From this ramshackle wooden building, the news went out that 'Pentecost has Come', a message that had been eagerly expected in churches throughout the world, particularly after the Welsh Revival of 1904–5.[18]

The end of the nineteenth century had been a period of intense religious fervour and there were numerous reports of miraculous healings. Speaking with tongues had become a coveted sign of possessing the Holy Spirit, as had the ability to heal. When young Evan Roberts felt the 'call' to ignite the Revival in Wales in 1904, his sister wrote of what happened when he came home one day unexpectedly:

> When Evan came home, Dan was lying on the couch looking very disheartened. Evan could not understand what was wrong, and then Dan told him he was losing his sight . . . and that a Llanelli specialist had told him there was no hope . . . [Evan] turned to Dan and said, 'You shall have your sight – the Lord has need of you.' Suddenly Dan regained his sight. A sort of miracle happened, and when he went to see the specialist, he marvelled, unable to explain what had happened.[19]

Pentecostal spirituality and teachings flowed from many sources in the Protestant chapels of this period, and from these emerged hundreds of independent Pentecostal Churches some quite small but others, like the Assemblies of God, with millions of members. A feature they shared was the emphasis they placed on personal conversion, baptism of the Holy Spirit, speaking in tongues (glossolalia), divine healing, preaching the Full Gospel message and the expectation of Christ's imminent return. Healings were a very prominent feature of the times and the Azusa Street Mission's paper, *Apostolic Faith*, was full of healing testimonials. In 1908 the lead article in a later publication, *Pentecost*, carried the headline, 'Broken Arm

Healed', and it was almost commonplace at meetings for members of the congregation to be slain by the spirit. This phenomenon, also known as resting in Jesus, was an early feature of the ministry of Maria Woodworth-Etter (1844–1924), an American evangelist who joined the Pentecostal movement in 1912.[20] She conducted huge, highly emotional healing rallies, where people would fall down and lie supine on the ground when she touched them.

Such behaviour is now quite acceptable in some churches and I have seen it happen at quite sedate gatherings of senior members of mainstream churches. Don Latham, a lay member of the Church of England, has experience of leading this type of service and describes an occasion where he was the principal speaker at a gathering of 300 Frenchmen. He felt inspired to speak to each man briefly, and wrote:

> The next day having delivered the talk, I invited men who wished for prayer to come forward – firstly from one block of the auditorium they all stood up and came forward. I got them into lines, and went forward to the first man. Without touching him I said 'Au nom de Jésus', and he fell backwards as the Holy Spirit came upon him. As I walked down the row, and spoke the name of Jesus it happened that way. Within ten minutes everyone, including the leaders who had been with me, had the same experience. There was no emotionalism, just peace and a strong smell of garlic.[21]

He describes a similar response, a few weeks later, at Hull University and again shortly afterwards at Swindon. Many people find such an experience helpful but others find it disturbing, particularly when it occurs in an emotionally fraught atmosphere. I remember discussing this with a young visitor to Coventry cathedral. She had been employed by a church in Scotland and had attended charismatic healing services there, which had disturbed her greatly. It was the sight of people falling down and convulsing, in the belief that they were being healed by the Holy Spirit, that upset her most and turned her from the Church. She still held to her 'core beliefs', but no longer wished to be involved with the Church as an institution. My friend John became disillusioned with the healing ministry after attending a charismatic mass in a Catholic church where the priest deliberately tried to make people fall backwards by exerting pressure on their foreheads.

A sociologist studied the effectiveness of healing in a Canadian settlement in the 1980s. He spent twelve months on the northeast coast of Newfoundland, in a village with 400 residents and two churches. One church was Pentecostal (PC) the other was not (NP), both were fundamentalist. The PC church provided a special healing service every Sunday in which the whole congregation participated. The approach to healing was much more muted in the NP church. The researcher found no evidence of a difference in the incidence of physical illness or physical healing in members of the two groups. He did, however, note that members of the Pentecostal church were less likely to report symptoms of emotional distress.

The study also provided a useful insight into the management and conduct of healing services within the churches. There was very little interest in healing within the NP church, but the PC church had regular healing services, which its congregation considered effective and important. The central part of the service was anointing with oil and the laying on of hands, acts which were performed by the pastor and elders, and carried out in an atmosphere of intense group support with stirring music, singing, dancing in the Spirit and speaking in tongues. Part of every Sunday service was set aside for this ritual, which involved the whole congregation: it would continue for over an hour and included the giving of testimonies.

Dancing in the Spirit was undertaken mainly by the men. They danced with frenetic, twisting movements, gyrating around the church before rolling on the floor for several minutes until eventually lying still. Then the other 'saints' gathered around the individual to hear the Spirit's message which he now uttered, usually in tongues. Women were more likely to give a testimony. The main themes of these testimonies were gratitude for being saved; gratitude for being healed; appeals for sinners in the community to be saved; and requests for help with personal and family problems. A typical testimony might begin:

> Precious Jesus, precious Jesus. I am glad to stand tonight and say I'm under the blood. Praise God for saving my soul when I was living in sin . . . last year I was sick, praise God I asked for healing and I felt the heat from his hands my friends. I stand here whole, praise the Lord.[22]

Requests for healing in the NP church were infrequent and always prefaced by the phrase, 'If it be your will . . . Heal me Lord.' There was little group support for healing in this church and its members could see no evidence of healings in the Pentecostal community. The finding that members of the Pentecostal church were less likely to experience emotional distress is interesting and, I think, only to be expected. The east coast of Canada is a bleak, desolate area, particularly in the winter, with little to stimulate the spirits of the inhabitants. I am sure that the cathartic affect of dancing in the Spirit must be very liberating for the men who live there.

Charismatic Movement

One direct consequence of the Pentecostal movement was the acceptance of charisma by mainstream churches in the 1950s, bringing healings, baptism of the Spirit and glossolalia with it. This development did not occur by chance or simply through the Power of the Holy Spirit; the groundwork had already been done by organizations such as The Order of St Luke and the Full Gospel Business Men's Fellowship International (FGBMFI). Demos Shakarian, a Californian dairy farmer, set up the FGBM-FI in 1951 with the aim of evangelizing and witnessing to non-Pentecostals. It soon established close links with many prominent, healing evangelists, notably Oral Roberts, who were campaigning in the United States and overseas. The importance of this link cannot be overemphasized, but the person most closely connected with the emergence of charisma was probably Agnes Sanford, the wife of an American Episcopalian priest.

Agnes became interested in healing early in her married life when it helped her through a severe depressive illness. In the 1930s she became involved with Camps Farthest Out (CFO), week-long camps in the United States, which her friend Glenn Clark organized for non-Pentecostal Christians. Like all the leading figures of CFO she taught and practised divine healing and when an Anglican priest, John Gaynor Banks, founded the Order of St Luke in 1947, she lent her enthusiasm and skills to that organization also. Most importantly she then opened, with her husband, the School of Pastoral Care where doctors, nurses and ministers of all religious denominations, were taught how to heal through faith and prayer. She also encouraged them to acquire the gift of tongues and introduced them to the idea of baptism in the Spirit. It was through these agencies that the mainstream Churches accepted the ethos behind Pentecostal teaching.

Comparisons are naturally drawn between the Pentecostal and Charismatic movements. The two obviously have much in common, particularly the emphasis on healing, speaking in tongues (and interpreting them) and baptism in the Spirit. It is said that in Britain there is a discernible socio-economic divide between the two movements, the Charismatics attending traditional Churches and the Pentecostals independent (often black) Churches, though this is not so evident in the rest of Europe and the United States. Perhaps more interesting is the observation that Pentecostal churches are quick to provide evidence of physical healing while Charismatic congregations are more focused on healing the inner being.[23]

Charisma is now to be found in many Roman Catholic parishes. The Catholic Church has always taught that healing of the inner person is a natural by-product of confession, the mass itself and the use of anointing as a healing sacrament, but the recent upsurge in interest in physical healing within the Church is remarkable. The hierarchy has supported many of the changes, but Rome has not approved all the new activities, particularly the healing rituals practised by some African bishops, notably Archbishop Emmanuel Milingo. The Congregation for the Doctrine of Faith continues to warn against mass hysteria and 'other excesses' but in general the Church is supportive of the new developments and a conference in Rome in November 2001 on *Prayer for Healing and the Charismatic Renewal of the Catholic Church* endorsed this attitude.[24]

Many charismatic leaders believe that the ministry of healing has come of age in Catholic parishes and is likely to have an even greater role in the daily life of the Church. How wonderful, they say, if after mass on a Sunday morning, anyone who wanted prayer at a difficult time in their life could find a few people who would spend some time praying with them. This is seen as a new field of pastoral care which will involve the laity as well as the priests. It is a practice that is also becoming acceptable in Anglican churches and I am told that the congregations tend to be larger when this ministry is available.

In recent years there has been an increasing readiness of retreat centres to include healing among the attractions they offer to their guests. This is in addition to the more usual provision of spiritual counselling in a quiet setting where one can reappraise one's life, or courses on painting, dance and music. Monastic communities now offer workshops on healing, aromatherapy, *Reiki*, reflexology, *Tai-chi chuan* and yoga. Some even offer an introduction to clowning, a most liberating activity, and the provision of these facilities is not limited to Catholic institutions; they are also available at Quaker centres and retreat houses run by the Anglican Church.

Chapter Six
Spiritual Healers (Christian)

There is no great mystery to healing. The body is wonderfully designed to heal itself and anyone can help it to do so with some measure of success. Perhaps its simplest expression is when a mother comforts a child who has fallen and hurt itself. She brings to the situation love, compassion and a desire to heal. The pain is eased by her concern and presence, helped perhaps by the simple words 'I'll kiss it better' and the kiss itself. But this innate ability can be greatly enhanced by training and practice, and this is true for both conventional and spiritual healers. Just as a paramedic is more useful than an untrained passerby at a road accident, someone who has acquired confidence and skill in spiritual healing can expect a more rewarding ministry than those who have pursued other interests.

In this chapter I concentrate on Christian healers, but a person does not need to have a particular religious faith to be an effective healer. In my profession, I find no difference in the effectiveness of Christian, Jewish or Muslim doctors, nor would I expect a Buddhist or Christian mother to have more success in comforting her child than a Hindu one. There are, of course, culturally based differences in the way people envisage healing and here, with the help of brief pen portraits, we'll see how seven twentieth-century Christian healers approached their task.

People of many religions regard Jesus of Nazareth as the archetypal healer *par excellence*. Christians see him in a special light but the healing resource he used – God's unconditional love – is available to everyone. Some people are able to tap this resource with greater ease than others and among these was the Capuchin Friar, Padre Pio of Pietrelcina (1887–1968). He was a most remarkable man who would obviously merit a place in this section but this aspect of his life's work has been dealt with in Chapter 3. Dorothy Kerin is included here. She was Padre Pio's English contemporary and in some ways her life resembled his. Both were sickly children, both were stigmatists who had visions of Christ and the Virgin Mary, and both had out-of-body experiences. Yet they were both practical people who

established hospitals/nursing homes – Padre Pio in Italy and Dorothy
Kerin in London and Kent. But we start with a man who was brought up in
the Welsh village where my daughter, Anna, now lives.

Rees Howells (1879–1950)

Intercessor.
Norman Grubb

Born in Brynamman, a Welsh mining village, Rees Howells left school at
the age of twelve to work in a tin-mill. He is best known as an intercessor,
one who pleads for another, but he was also an inspiring evangelist, a missionary in Africa and a notable healer. One friend described him as 'the
biggest hearted Christian I ever met' and another that 'he was the most
wonderful missionary I had read of'. Fortunately, his life-history is well documented by Norman Grubb, who tells us that his healings involved much
prayer and fasting.[1]

Howells was a strong, well-built man who enjoyed boxing and physical
activities, yet he was conscious of God's presence from an early age, and
preferred the Welsh mountains, chapels and prayer meetings to the big
town delights available in nearby Swansea. He was also an ambitious
young man who wanted to be wealthy, so he emigrated to Pittsburgh when
he was twenty-two. There he joined a local church and never missed a
prayer meeting. At that time he almost died from typhoid fever, a close
encounter with death that frightened him and may have prepared him for
the conversion experience that soon followed. This took place in a small
Methodist chapel during a service conducted by the evangelist Maurice
Reuben, a Christian Jew.

In later years Howells spoke of this event as his 'spiritual birthday' and
'the most outstanding day of my life' and he never forgot the debt he owed
to the Jewish people. During the Nazi period, he provided a home for young
Jewish refugees and when the Italian government declared that every Jew
had to leave the country within six months, he began a continuing ministry
of intercessory prayer for the Jewish people. His thoughts also turned to the
possibility of the Jews returning to Palestine, and he would say, 'I have a
great burden for these people and I want God to lay their burden on me. . .
I am longing to help God's people to return to their own land.'[2]

Rees Howells healed by intercessory prayer. He made an interesting distinction between a 'prayer warrior' and an 'intercessor'. In his view prayer
warriors can pray for a thing to be done without requiring that the answer
should come through themselves, and they are not bound to continue in
the prayer until it has been answered. The intercessor has a greater respon-

sibility, he has to gain the objective and is never free until it has been achieved. An intercessor will go to any lengths for the prayer to be answered through themselves personally, but once a position of intercession has been gained, tested and proved, the intercessor can claim all the blessings at that level of intercession, whenever it is God's will for them to do so. He would often speak of 'the gained position of intercession' and say that once the inner wrestlings and groanings have run their course and the obedience fulfilled, then the weak vessel is clothed with authority by the Holy Ghost and can speak the word of deliverance. He likened the situation to a geometrical theorem where once a person has learnt the propositions, he can use them as a basis for future work and does not need to cover the same ground twice.[3]

Howells returned to Wales in 1904, the year of the great Welsh Revival. He was much involved in this movement but also found paid employment in a local coal mine. The first person to approach him for healing was a young woman suffering from tuberculosis. His attempt to heal her created a lot of local interest, and though initially there was some improvement, the woman died. Her funeral was attended by hundreds of mourners and was conducted by a minister who had been critical of Howells' involvement, and he made his position clear in the biblical text he chose for his sermon: Job 13: 1–5 (King James version).

> But ye are forgers of lies, ye are all physicians of no value. Oh that ye would altogether hold your peace! and it should be your wisdom.

It was a difficult time for Howells.

A few months later Howells was asked to visit a man in the village who was dying. The wife was distraught as there were ten children to support, and her husband was already unconscious. Howells returned the next day to inform the wife that her husband would not die and promised that he himself would support her and the children if the father died. The man recovered. Rees was also asked to visit the sister of the woman who had died of tuberculosis. She was dangerously ill after childbirth and the doctor offered no hope that she would survive. The family's immediate concern was to know God's will for her. Rees could not give an instant reply but as he walked home he felt the word of God come to him, and he was so sure that she would be healed that he returned to tell them the good news and the woman's condition immediately began to improve.

The healing of Uncle Dick was particularly notable. Uncle Dick lived in Pentwyn, on the Black Mountains, in the grandparents' old home and he had been an invalid for many years. One day, the Holy Spirit informed Rees that his uncle was to be healed and would walk again. On his next visit to Pentwyn, he told his uncle what he had heard and the old man went into the garden to pray. He returned with his face radiant. 'Yes,' he said, 'I am to be healed in four and a half months, that will be on May 15th.' Soon the news became the talk of the district, but shortly afterwards Uncle Dick became ill and spent the next four weeks in bed. During this time the Holy Spirit told the family not to pray for healing and that Dick should prepare himself for the work that he would undertake after being healed, which would be on Whitsunday. Dick had been told by the Spirit that he would be healed at 5 am and that he was to walk to chapel, which he had not done for thirty years. He slept until 5 am woke up and found himself fit and well. His family and friends were amazed. During the next five years Dick acted as an honorary minister, visiting every house in the neighbourhood and opening many prayer meetings. He remained well and active until the day of his death.

Rees Howells and his wife spent six years in Africa as missionaries, returning to Wales at Christmas 1920. While in Africa he had a severe bout of malaria, which did not respond to treatment, his condition deteriorated so rapidly that his wife, in her distress, had to go outside to pray for him. While he was alone in the house the Holy Spirit said to him, 'Why don't you ask the Father to heal you?' Rees thought that he had, but the Spirit said to him, 'You didn't ask believing.' After this reprimand, he said, 'I just turned over in bed and in that moment was healed. I wondered if my wife would know it. Would she have lost her burden?' The moment she re-entered the room, his wife realized what had happened and said, '"You have been healed" and I laughed and told her about it.' He never had malaria again.

The great pandemic of Spanish influenza which caused millions of deaths throughout the world spread to Africa at about this time. The disease eventually reached Rusitu in East Africa where the Howells were based, and a number of people on the mission station became ill. A few days later, the local chief sent a deputation to ask if anyone had died from the 'flu. 'No,' Rees replied. 'Have you had any deaths?' 'Yes, many,' they said. The deputation returned a few days later but there had still been no deaths, and Rees felt moved to say that no one would die on the station, and that anyone who wished to join them would be made welcome. Dozens of people came and even though the epidemic raged for three months no one died on the station, though some, including his wife, became desperately ill. Later, he was able to say: 'How I praised God for my personal guide.'[4]

His fame lives on. In 1999 my wife and I visited Santiago de Compostela with a group of people from Essex. The group included a lady who had spent her childhood in East Africa where her parents had been missionaries. The name Rees Howells surfaced in the conversation and to my great surprise she had heard many firsthand reports of the big impact he had made in African society eighty years earlier.

J. Cameron Peddie (1887-1968)

Cameron Peddie was a Scottish Presbyterian minister. He was a modest person of outstanding character, and the man mainly responsible for the establishment of a 'healing ministry' in the Church of Scotland. A 'country boy' who obtained his education through scholarships, he was ordained a minister in 1917. Three years later, he decided that he would do better work as a doctor and enrolled as a medical student at Aberdeen university, but then he received a 'call' to another church, a summons he felt he could not refuse.

In 1929, he moved to the Gorbals in Glasgow and here he felt that his life's work really began. The Gorbals was a very tough area with a large, lawless constituency organized into about thirty gangs, each with some 200 members. The most notorious gang – the South Side Stickers – had committed six murders before Peddie moved into the area, and soon afterwards the gangs had a pitched battle outside his church. A group of local businessmen asked him to deal with the problem, so instead of going away for his summer vacation he stayed at home, got to know the men[5] and persuaded the South Side Stickers to reform as a club with their gang boss as the club leader. This move had such an impact locally that within two years there were thirty clubs in the Gorbals. To help the clubs, Peddie obtained possession of vacant shops and factories and organized work schemes – including a firewood factory, an advertising agency, a vinegar bottling factory and a knitwear cooperative for the women – which gave the unemployed members a certain measure of independence and self-respect.

In 1942, his interest in medical work was rekindled whilst he was a patient in a Glasgow hospital. There, he met a young man who was being sent home to die, and he resolved to examine more seriously Christ's commission to His church to 'preach the Gospel and heal the sick'. When he returned home, a Jewish friend, whose wife had cancer of the throat, asked him on three separate occasions if it would be right for him to take her to a spiritualist healer. Twice he replied 'No' but on the third occasion he said, 'Yes, for goodness sake take your wife to the woman. If she does her no good, she will do her no harm.'

The visit was such a great success that Peddie decided to investigate further and made an appointment for his own wife and son to see the healer. Both had chronic disabilities: the son being asthmatic and Mrs Peddie having long-standing pain due to fibrositis. All three were impressed by the healer, by her sincerity, attitude and kindness. Her own son had died in infancy and she had then asked God to use her for this healing work. Several years passed by without any indication that this was to be her vocation, then suddenly she found that she could heal when under the control of a discarnate spirit. In describing the consultation. Peddie said that the healer sat down on a chair and

> Gradually the expression on her face changed and the features seemed to alter, taking on an eastern appearance. She was under trance. 'Good morning' said the spirit and she offered up one of the most beautiful prayers I have ever heard. We felt ourselves in the presence of an angel – certainly not a devil.[6]

She treated Mrs Peddie and her son for about half an hour each: and following this ministration the son's condition improved greatly and the wife's pain disappeared completely. Peddie was so impressed that he decided – expressing it as a solemn covenant with God – that he would prepare himself to become a suitable vehicle for the Holy Spirit to use in the same way. Each night for five years he spent the hour from 11 pm to midnight alone in his sanctuary with God, offering every bodily organ by name and every cell in his body to be recreated for this work. He adopted the same approach to his thoughts and feelings, praying that every memory, thought, imagination, will and his Ego itself be renewed. He followed this spiritual discipline with the intention of becoming 'a medium of the spirit that was in Christ Jesus'.

Eventually, he started to look for a sign that would convince him that he was fully prepared for the task ahead: this came on the 17 May 1947, exactly thirty years to the hour after his ordination. At that moment he felt himself gripped by a strange, benevolent power that filled him with an indescribable sense of happiness. It seemed to draw him out of his body, and though he did not know whether he was in the body or out of it, he experienced such bliss and joy that his eyes filled with tears and he cried like a child. He felt as if he was the Prodigal Son being reunited with the Father and he knew quite simply that: 'God is and that He rewards all who diligently seek Him.'

There were times later when he worried in case the sense of power was of the Devil and he asked to be reassured that it was truly of God. This reassurance came in May 1948 when he was praying. He saw that his right hand was becoming smaller and bruised as though it had been hammered. Then a large nail appeared between the roots of the first two fingers, and blood started to trickle on to the palms and over the wrists. He could not recall how long the vision lasted but he was now sure of his mission; the only uncertainty was where to begin.

This impasse was resolved when he visited a journalist friend and his wife. She was seriously ill with heart failure, she was also deaf in one ear and had rheumatic problems. During the visit she said: 'Mr Peddie, 1 believe you could heal me if you liked!' to which he replied, 'I believe I could.' When he returned a few days later, she was lying in bed covered with blankets, and as he laid his hands on her, he had an experience, which was never repeated. He had a vision in which she was 'lying in a bath of light so indescribable in its beauty and brilliance, that I can call it only the Glory of God'. She lay in the light throughout the half-hour that he ministered to her, and he believes something similar happens whenever people minister in the name and power of Jesus Christ. He never gave a more effective healing. Within half an hour the pains had gone and the hearing in the 'deaf' ear was better than in the healthy one.[7]

When people received healing from Cameron Peddie, they sometimes felt as if sea breezes were blowing new life into them. This sensation was reported so frequently that his daughter called it 'Daddy's sea breezes', and a visiting minister from Canada, the Revd Allan Old, mentioned it when describing his own healing. This, he said, began with a chat, then he sat on a chair and Peddie, who stood about two feet in front of him, placed his hands close to his head and slowly lowered them without touching his body. Then he placed his hands on Old's back and prayed, first aloud then in silence. Old wrote:

> The interesting thing was that as he very slowly lowered his hands in front of me a fresh breeze seemed to come from them . . . And the breeze had a fragrance, my wife and I thought to be very similar to that of pine wood. This fragrance came from small beads of oil which appeared on the palms of his hands after Mr Peddie started to work.

He also says that although he had been treated by several of the world's best known healers, only Cameron Peddie had been able to help his back at all.[8]

Peddie believed that healing was an integral part of the Christian minister's duty. He felt this very strongly and was largely responsible for starting a healing ministry in the Scottish Churches. The Christian Fellowship of Healing (Scotland), as it is now called, is a group of Christians from many denominations who are involved with the healing ministry. Its original purpose was to support clergy in the practice of laying on of hands and in the organization of intercessory groups. In the early days, Peddie would travel hundreds of miles to help a colleague with an intractable healing problem: he accompanied them on visits to the sick and at healing services so they could gain the confidence and expertise to manage alone.

Dorothy Kerin (1889–1963)

She brings them Christ.
Johanna Ernest

Dorothy Kerin had an enormous impact on the healing ministry in the Church of England. She had herself been healed at the age of twenty-two when she was seriously ill, and the healing ministry which she later developed was so successful that it is likely to have been a major factor in the decision in 1953 by the English Archbishops to set up a Commission on Divine Healing. This led in 1983 to the appointment of Bishop Morris Maddocks as the first national co-ordinator of the Church of England's Healing Ministry, and to the publication in 2000 of the Church of England's major report, *A Time to Heal*.

Dorothy Kerin was a frail, energetic woman who said that anything she achieved was done through the Grace of God. She established centres for spiritual healing and recuperation in London, adopted nine babies, accepted many invitations to speak, both at home and abroad, which she always did without notes, and above all learnt the necessity of being obedient to God's will. The mainstay of her healing ministry was quite simply the imperative of abandoning the human will to Christ. She was a remarkable healer, yet a friend could say of her:

> Many people have been cured of sickness, often of incurable sickness, through the prayers and ministrations of Dorothy Kerin. But she never, never, I am sure, primarily brings healing. She brings them Christ.[9]

Support for this assessment comes from an observation made by her friend, Bishop Cuthbert Bardsley. A few months before she died, Dorothy was conducting a healing service at All Saints Church, Leamington Spa and, as she ascended the pulpit, the bishop prayed for her to be given strength. He wrote:

> Then a remarkable thing happened. Over Dorothy's face gradually appeared the face of Christ, until it was quite clear. For a few moments the beloved face of Our Lord was there, and then gradually faded away, and Dorothy's face returned. I had clearly been shown that Christ was already there to strengthen her, and she carried on bravely to the end of the service.[10]

Dorothy Kerin was born in London. Her father, the son of an army surgeon, died when she was twelve years old and this loss affected her deeply. She had a happy childhood but after her father's death she had a long succession of illnesses, including diphtheria, pneumonia and tuberculosis. She was a permanent invalid for almost five years then, in December 1911, the doctors diagnosed tubercular meningitis. On Sunday, 4 February 1912, she received the Blessed Sacrament and as the priest came towards her with the chalice, she saw a golden light radiating from the cup enveloping the priest, and she felt a wonderful sense of God's Presence in which she was carried out of the body to a heavenly realm.

By 18 February 1912, she was blind, deaf, emaciated and semiconscious, and her physician left the house that day, saying her death was imminent. Then she had a remarkable experience. She found herself surrounded by a great light, which radiated from an angel, who told her that her sufferings were over and that she was to get up and walk. She opened her eyes and found herself lying in bed, surrounded by family and friends, a total of sixteen people, waiting for her to die. She told them that she was quite well and asked for her dressing gown which she put on, then got out of bed unaided, placed her hand on the light and walked. Later she wrote:

> This led me out of the room and though I had not walked for five years, I now walked quite steadily, and felt so well and strong that I might not have been ill at all. Soon after, I felt hungry and asked for food which they brought me in a feeding cup. That I refused to take and went to the larder and helped myself to a meal of meat and pudding which I ate without any pain or discomfort. Later I returned to bed and slept until the following morning. When I got up my family were amazed at the change in my bodily appearance. Instead of looking like a skeleton, my body appeared normal. I was quite plump, my bones being covered with firm healthy flesh – all this in the space of twelve hours.[11]

The Evening News reported the healing on 20 February. *The Daily Chronicle*, in its account on the 21 February, included a statement by her GP, Dr Norman FRCS, which stated:

> Had I read of it I certainly should not have believed it. She is well, but how she got better, I do not know.[12]

Three days later, Dr Edwin Ash, a consultant physician, invited Dorothy to stay at his home. She was there for six weeks whilst he carried out various medical tests, and during this time she had another vision. On 11 March, she awoke to see a great light at the foot of her bed and in it the image of a beautiful lady holding a lily: the lady came close and told her that she would heal many sick people and comfort the sorrowing. When she awoke in the morning, she could still smell the scent of the lily.[13] By this time her recovery had caused so much public interest that she issued a statement in the *London Budget* on the 30 June. In it she made the following points.

- That the healing came directly from God without intermediary agency.
- She had not prayed to be healed; her prayer was that she would be happy in doing what God might will.
- Prayer is the tonic that creates an appetite for things of the spirit.
- Christ is as alive today as when he was upon earth.
- That power unlimited, sublime and free, is within reach of us all.[14]

Dorothy now realized that God was calling her to the healing ministry, but there was a long period of preparation before she took up her vocation. She had further visions, and also out-of-body experiences in which she found herself in no-man's-land on the Western Front ministering to wounded and dying soldiers. Then, on 8 December 1915, the stigmata began to appear on her body. These marks of Christ's crucifixion appeared first in her left hand, the other lesions appearing over the next few days and, during this time, Dorothy experienced much suffering and inner desolation. The wounds remained open for several days and were seen by a number of people, including eleven who signed statements attesting to their authenticity.[15] The marks remained visible for several years afterwards.

Between 1915 and 1929, she lived with the Revd Dr Langford-James and his wife as their adopted daughter. He became her spiritual director[16] and she took the threefold vow of poverty, chastity and obedience, a decision which she later regretted. In 1929, she received a gift of money and this, with the support of a few friends, enabled her to open her first Home of Healing in London. She rented and renovated a building, which she called Chapel House, and accepted all those in need of help free of charge. The demand for places was so great that it became necessary to enlarge the building, and she continued this work throughout the Second World War, acquiring more properties to cope with the number of people turning to her for care so that by 1945 she owned seven properties and had adopted nine children.

Later she founded a new healing centre in Burrswood, Kent, where she sought to integrate the best of medical, nursing and spiritual care so that every need of her patients was addressed. In 1959 she built the Church of Christ the Healer as a focal point for the spiritual life of Burrswood. Here the Eucharist is offered daily for healing throughout the world, and public healing services are held regularly for visitors, patients and guests.[17]

Dorothy's healing ministry is based on the 'Gethsemane' approach to prayer. This is quite different from that of Rees Howells and those other 'prayer warriors' who strive to storm the gates of heaven to achieve what they want. Her attitude may be summed up in Christ's words 'Not my will but Yours be done' and this is the basis of her 'Little Way of Prayer':

> Let us by an act of will place ourselves in the presence of our Divine Lord, and with an act of faith ask that He will empty us of self and of all desire save that His Most Blessed Will be done, and that it will illumine our hearts and minds. We can then gather together ourselves and all those for whom our prayers have been asked and hold them silently up to Him, making no special request – neither asking nor beseeching – but just resting, with them, in Him, desiring nothing but that Our Lord may be glorified in all. In this most simple way of approach He does make known His Most Blessed Will for us. For so He giveth Himself to His beloved in quietness.

David Flagg, chaplain at Burrswood, calls the concept behind this prayer a resting theology, and Bishop Morris Maddocks could truly say that 'this contemplative approach to healing prayer, resting in the Lord and seeking only His will was indeed one of Dorothy's legacies to the praying church'.[18]

Finally, on 27 June 1958, she set out her vision of integrated medicine quite clearly in a letter to *The Church Times*:

> If our Church is to live it must restore its ministry of healing . . . and it will find, as I have in thirty years of work in the ministry of healing, that religion and medicine work harmoniously hand in hand. I have never experienced any conflict and have found the medical profession most eager to accept spiritual co-operation.

Hilda Ingram

Coventry housewife

It is important to remember that most healers are not famous, they are ordinary people who practise quietly in their own neighbourhoods content with the recognition they receive from those whom they help. Some belong to mainstream churches, others do not, but they all strive to reduce the burden of human distress. Hilda Ingram was one such healer and she is included partly as a representative of this unsung group, but mainly because she was known to David Yates, a friend who told me her story.

Hilda was a housewife who developed her healing skills whilst caring for her husband during his long illness. Although healing can be physically tiring, and in some ways a lonely ministry, Hilda received a lot of support from the Bishop of Coventry, Cuthbert Bardsley, a friend and supporter of Dorothy Kerin. He dedicated a room in Hilda's house as a healing chapel and appointed a local priest, Harry Puntis, to be her personal chaplain. Hilda was a great talker: some people found this irritating as she would chat away for twenty minutes or so before laying hands on the sick person, but this was a critical period of the session as it enabled her to get in tune with the patient and discover what their real problems were, before she ministered to them. What is more, she shared this knowledge with the patient before attempting the healing.

Hilda was very open in her ministry. She was prepared to heal people in their own homes, in hospitals or at church services. For many years she held a monthly service in her local church, but this always left her exhausted as she empathized with the sufferer's condition to such an extent that if the patient was in pain then Hilda would feel it herself. The amount of time she spent in laying-on of hands depended on the situation. At a church service, with twenty people wanting relief only about five minutes could be given to each one. In the privacy of the home, she would spend about twenty minutes touching the entire body from top to toe, with the patient experiencing this as an intense heat which radiated from her hands right to the centre of the body.

Hilda's story is not an entirely happy one. She had the Bishop's support, but there were varying levels of enthusiasm for her ministry in the diocese and the attitude of newly appointed priests sometimes did not help. She began to feel that her role in the parish church was being diminished but despite such setbacks she continued to heal people in their homes and in hospitals when asked. Her effectiveness may be assessed from the following reports.

Case 1: A young girl was in hospital with meningitis. She had been coma-tose for three weeks and the nurses were sure that even if she regained consciousness she would be brain-damaged. The Revd Harry Puntis asked twelve members of his congregation to pray together in church whilst Hilda was ministering to the child in hospital. To everyone's surprise the child immediately regained consciousness, sat up in bed and made a full recovery with no mental impairment. She is now a married woman with two children.

Case 2: Mike was a thirty-five years-old, married man with two daughters when he was admitted to hospital with an inoperable cancer of the gut. After he had been discharged, David Yates asked him if he would like to meet a lady with a gift of healing, to which he replied: 'I am an atheist, but I will try anything once.' Hilda always said that she could never cure cancer but she could relieve pain, so she visited Mike and placed her hands all over his body for about twenty minutes. Later, Mike said that he felt like the 'ReadyBrek' advert, in which a young boy is portrayed as surrounded by a vibrant red glow. To this Hilda replied: 'Mike you are surrounded by the love of Jesus.' She continued to minister to him at home until he became so ill that he had to be readmitted to hospital. Every time he was conscious, he asked to see Hilda and she would visit him. He also asked the vicar to visit and pray with him, and he became a believer. David Yates said, 'It was a tremendous experience for all of us.'

Case 3: Dennis was blind and dependent on his wife. She was admitted to hospital for an operation on her toe but there were complications and she was transferred to another hospital in a coma. David Yates phoned Dennis and arranged for Hilda to visit the wife. On the appointed day she was unconscious when they arrived in the ward, and David and a friend went to pray in the hospital chapel while Hilda ministered at the bedside. They returned to the ward twenty minutes later to find the patient sitting up and wide awake. She made a full recovery and lived another seven years before dying from cancer.

Case 4: A young mother was confined to bed with severe backache. A spinal operation seemed inevitable when her vicar, the Revd Laurence Mortimer, asked Hilda to help. She visited and laid her hands upon the young woman who recovered almost immediately and was soon leading a normal life. She had her third baby twelve months later and there was no recurrence of the back problem.

Hilda died suddenly at home some months after her son was killed in a road traffic accident. By then her fame had spread beyond Coventry. The Revd Eric Fisher knew her and in his book *Healing Miracles*,[19] writes:

> After one service Mrs Ingram showed me her hands. They were covered with a slight film of oil, quite apparent and distinctive.

He goes on to compare the appearance of this oil with the healing oil mentioned by St James when he wrote: 'Is there anyone who is ill? He should send for the church elders, who will pray for him and rub oil on him in the name of the Lord.'[20] A Canadian clergyman noticed the same phenomenon when he received healing from the Revd Cameron Peddie. Describing the incident, Peddie wrote:

> Suddenly he said to me, 'Peddie your hands are oily. You are anointing me with oil.' I lifted my hands and we both looked at them. All over there was a thin film of oil with solitary globules here and there. It was no illusion: it was a physical reality. In a little while, he said, 'Peddie, the oil is perfumed', and so it was. It had a strange, sweet pleasant aroma.[21]

Agnes Sanford (1897–1982)

She is perhaps more responsible than anyone else for renewing the healing ministry in mainline churches.
Francis MacNutt[22]

Agnes Sanford was born in China of American parents. Her formative years were happy and spent mainly in China where her father was a Presbyterian minister. She married an Episcopalian missionary and soon after their marriage he decided to move to New Jersey, so they spent most of their married life in the United States. At first she was very unhappy there, but it was during this period that her interest in healing began. The defining moment occurred when her son, Jack, had a painful infection of the ear and Hollis Colwell, an Episcopalian priest who happened to be in the house at the time, placed his hands over the boy's ears and prayed. The child closed his eyes and went to sleep. When he awoke his temperature was normal and the pain had gone.

Agnes felt so depressed and suicidal that she made an appointment to see Hollis Colwell at his house. After talking for a while he placed his hands on her head and prayed for the healing of her mental state. This act was crucial for Agnes. She was quite sure that if he had just counselled her and not prayed, she would have committed suicide. Instead, she felt as if the heavens had been opened and 'great waves of joy' flooded into her so that she 'sang and shouted at the top of [her] voice all the way home'.[23] When she saw Colwell next, he advised her to take up creative writing. This was something she had always wanted to do but never tried. Later, she was to give similar advice to many people, encouraging them to undertake some activity which they had secretly longed to do but had never attempted. She also started to use the Jesus prayer – the silent repetition of the words 'Lord Jesus Christ, Son of God, have mercy on me a sinner' – but changed the words slightly, so that the prayer became 'Lord Jesus Christ, Son of God, fill me with Thy life'. This version is much more appropriate for the depressed who might find the words 'fill me with your love' equally helpful as a supplication.

Following her healing, Agnes felt that she had become a new person. She started to experiment with prayer and healing, and eventually felt sufficiently confident to visit a hospital and pray for a parishioner's son who was desperately ill with streptococcal septicaemia before antibiotics had been discovered. She was terrified when she went into the hospital ward, but at the bedside she felt perfectly calm. The child was aware of what was happening and three days later was able to return home cured.[24]

Her healing ministry developed gradually over the years. In his assessment of her work, Professor Glen Clark wrote:

> She has tried and studied every form of healing that has ever been known. Never have I met one who combined the metaphysical and the sacramental approach as she does. I have never met anyone more Christ-centred nor anyone more church-centred and yet utterly unconcerned about the creed or lack of creed of those that she ministers to.[25]

Her approach combined great spiritual awareness with a deep understanding of human psychology. She recognized the healing power of the sacraments, including sacramental confession, yet believed that the sick should seek healing even if they had no overt faith. In such instances, her approach would be along these lines:

1. She would explain that there is a healing energy within the individual and also in the outside world, sometimes called 'nature', and that a

person could receive more of this if they ask.
2. The person to ask is God, but if you have no knowledge of God, you can ask for His help anyway.
3. Just say, 'Whoever you are, or whatever you are, come into me now and help nature to heal me.'[26]

Agnes was closely associated with three healing organizations. The first was Camps Farthest Out (CFO), which was founded in the 1930s by Glen Clark to help people develop their full potential in a Christian environment of faith. All the leading figures in CFO taught and practised divine healing through prayer, at a time when this was still regarded with suspicion. Later, Agnes became involved with the International Order of St Luke the Physician which was founded by the Revd John Gaynor Banks in 1947, and which has been described as 'the most prominent advocate of spiritual healing in the Episcopal Church'.[27] Her most important work, however, was with the School of Pastoral Care (SPC), which she set up in 1956 with her husband, Ted. Together they made a perfect team, possibly because they had such different personalities.

The aim of the SPC was to teach ministers aspects of the Christian faith that were not covered in theological colleges, in particular, healing of the body, mind and soul through faith and prayer. Seminars at the school lasted five days: they were open to doctors, nurses and ministers of religion, those in positions of leadership who, once they had acquired the ability to heal by the power of prayer, would be able to help so many more people.

It soon became obvious that all the trainees needed personal counselling, confession and prayer themselves, and this became part of the course. Such intimate matters were always handled individually, never in a group setting. In order to maintain harmony, there was only one period of questions and general discussion each day. This was called the 'hymn sing and question period' and was designed so that the heat could be taken out of confrontations. If any questions tended to be aggressive or the discussions time-wasting, the leader would say, 'Now who would like to suggest a hymn?' and so turn the feeling of the meeting to one of peace. The course included a 'prayer clinic' for the healing of trivial complaints. In this session participants were encouraged to reveal some minor indisposition and ask someone, who was inexperienced in healing, to lay hands on them.

Also at the SPC, Agnes encouraged people to be baptised in the Spirit and to speak in tongues. She did this very discreetly and Ted was never involved in this aspect of her ministry. She also saw the need to heal ancestral memories, work later undertaken by Dr Kenneth McAll when he began the Family Tree Ministry in the 1970s. It is of interest that both were born and lived for many years in China where it is believed that the ancestors play a continuing, significant role in everyday life.

Dr Kenneth McAll (1910-2001)

Japanese prisoner and psychiatrist.

Kenneth McAll had an unusual healing ministry. Born in China of missionary parents, he went to school at Eltham College, England, qualified in medicine at Edinburgh University and returned to China with a young Canadian wife in 1937. He was appointed superintendent at a hospital in Siaochang, in north China, the only centre providing western medicine to a population of ten million people in an area the size of Wales. Eric Liddell, the Scottish missionary who featured in the film *Chariots of Fire*, worked closely with him at the hospital.

Siaochang was not a peaceful place. The continuing Sino-Japanese conflict made life difficult and the hospital staff were expected to visit villagers in this war-torn area. On one occasion McAll had a strange experience. He was walking alone in the open country, and heading for a nearby village, when he became aware of someone behind him, who told him not to go to that particular village but to another where the need was greater. He followed the advice and when he reached the fence, the gate was opened and he was pulled inside. The villagers asked him why he had come to them, and he now realized that he was alone and, even more surprisingly, that the voice had spoken to him in English. He was told that there had been a local skirmish and that several wounded men had been brought to the village who needed his surgical skills. He was also told that the village he had intended to visit was occupied by Japanese soldiers. Later he wrote:

> I knew that it was Jesus who had appeared to me. My mocking tolerance of the implicit belief of the Chinese in ghosts and the spirit world was gone . . . and I realized that my daily prayer for protection had been dramatically answered.[28]

Together with his wife and young daughter, McAll was imprisoned by the Japanese during the Second World War. When he returned to England in 1945 he weighed just 8 stone. For some years, he practised as a GP, then specialized in psychiatry, though he never obtained any formal psychiatric qualifications. By this time he was convinced that many sick people were troubled by entities in the spirit world and that these disturbed spirits needed to be helped. He advanced the idea that many illnesses, such as anorexia nervosa, alcoholism, diabetes and the psychoses, were caused by 'lost souls', the unmourned dead who needed help, and that this was best provided by means of a Christian ritual, the Eucharist. Later in life he expressed surprise at this development in his thinking, saying: 'At one stage of my Christian life I felt we could not pray for the dead since judgement came immediately after death.'[29]

What he was advocating, of course, is the Requiem Mass of the Roman Catholic tradition, a suggestion that would have been anathema to the young McAll with his Scottish, Protestant missionary background. He now formed the Family Tree Ministry (FTM), an organization that he registered as a charity:

> For the benefit of the public at large and to the honour and glory of God for the promotion of Christian Healing in particular by the healing of the Family Tree through the Eucharist as pioneered by Dr Robert Kenneth McAll.

His wife, Dr Frances McAll, later defined its purpose equally succinctly when she wrote:

> The FTM exists to promote the Christian healing approach pioneered by Dr McAll. Many mental and some physical diseases may result from past family trauma, e.g. suicide or abortion. Healing follows the committal of the unmourned or unrecognized individual to God.[30]

People attending a FTM healing service are asked to compile a family tree and identify the family members for whom prayer is required. These may include the living and the dead, but a particular emphasis is placed on the needs of babies who were aborted, miscarried or stillborn, people who have committed suicide, and drug and alcohol abusers. The importance given to babies who have died in the womb is noteworthy as this is an area that was totally neglected by the Christian Churches until the 1980s. Then with a growing awareness of the importance of bereavement care and the new insights provided by psychiatrists, such as Colin Murray Parkes, hospital chaplains began to hold services for the aborted and stillborn, and in 1985, the Roman Catholic Church authorized a prayer for the aborted foetus, and in 1980 one for the stillborn child.

McAll recognized four key stages in the healing Eucharist:

1. The importance of the Lord's prayer. Here the emphasis is on deliverance and protection. 'Deliver us from Evil' carries the expectation that, through the communion wine, 'Jesus Christ should cleanse the blood lines of the living and the dead of all that blocks healthy life, especially by breaking any hereditary seals and curses and by casting out any evil spirits'.
2. The importance of forgiveness. The dead must be forgiven if we are to help them at the Eucharist, and we must ask for their forgiveness too. Forgiveness also means a shared love.
3. The bearing of witness to Christ's death and resurrection. In accepting the sacraments we share them, in our hearts, with those for whom we pray.

4. The final blessing. At this point the focus shifts from the needs of the dead to those of the living.[31] McAll says that at the Eucharist:

> We should always have specific intentions. Perhaps 1 per cent for ourselves, 99 per cent for others. Our prayers should be spoken aloud, shared with others we trust especially family members . . . To say them aloud makes the whole objective and takes the symptoms outside the patient, who can now hear and consciously cathect the situation.[32]

The Family Tree Ministry also teaches that certain places need healing. Its members do this by praying and celebrating the Eucharist at sites that have witnessed great tragedy and horror, such as battlefields, concentration camps and places where people have committed suicide. I heard Kenneth McAll speak on a number of occasions, but one of my clearest recollections is of attending the FTM conference at Walsingham. The church was packed for the Eucharist, and as the people prayed aloud for aborted babies and other family members, there was an unusual ripple of noise in that normally quiet church, and afterwards some participants claimed to have been reunited with their loved ones during the service.[33] I found the occasion was more emotionally charged than I had expected, but it was cathartic – I should probably describe it as healing, as I was able to unload some of the griefs and sense of guilt that I had accumulated during a medical career which had witnessed many deaths, miscarriages and suicides.

Oral Roberts (1918–)

King of the Faith Healers.
American Magazine

Oral Roberts was one of the most prominent religious leaders of the twentieth century. He was also one of the most controversial: people either adored him or despised him, depending on their reaction to his work, which covered three different fields. He was a passionate advocate of 'healing' as a Christian ministry, gave dynamic leadership and publicity to the Pentecostal and charismatic movements after the Second World War, and was one of the first to see how the media, particularly television, could be used to spread the Christian message to a much wider audience.[34]

Of mixed Celtic and Amerindian parentage, Roberts was born in Oklahoma where his father was a Pentecostal preacher. He was ordained in the Pentecostal Holiness Church at the age of eighteen, founded the Oral Roberts University in Tulsa in 1967 and, whilst remaining highly esteemed by Pentecostals, joined the United Methodist Church in 1968. During the late 1940s and 1950s, he was a leading figure among the American revivalists who took the Pentecostal gospel of healing and deliverance around the world. He conducted meetings in chapels, tents and in the open air, but from 1968 Roberts presented his message mainly through the media. He did this by means of a weekly television programme, his own radio station and a mass circulation monthly magazine.

Roberts was a powerful preacher in his heyday. His primary aim was the saving of lost souls and there would always be a call for repentance and salvation in his services. After the Salvation Call, a healing line would form and his healing ministry would begin: then he would exercise his skill in discerning and naming demons. Of this early ministry, his associate Dr Sproull wrote:

> It is amazing to see the people set free from demon spirits. Their faces shine, their eyes sparkle and frequently their entire body is visibly shaken. Sometimes while the demon spirits are being cast out by the power of faith in God, the demons throw the captives on the floor where they lie apparently lifeless until God's servant reaches down, saying 'Rise in the name of the Lord and be made whole.' They spring to their feet with new life and joy. The entire audience is powerfully moved for it is evident to all that the miraculous has taken place before their very eyes.[35]

Other Christian groups were much more sceptical and often hotly disputed the claims of miraculous healings associated with these meetings. A Protestant sect, the Churches of Christ, was one of the most vigorous critics of Roberts' methods and, when his healing crusades were advertised, would challenge him to a debate and offer rewards of $1,000 for documentary evidence that a healing had actually occurred. Typically, they placed the following notice in a Florida newspaper after a Roberts campaign in 1955.

> In view of the fact that a revival campaign has just concluded in which claims were made both over the radio and through the mails that many have been healed . . . the Churches of Christ felt compelled to take this means of bringing out the fact that NOT ONE SINGLE CASE OF MIRACULOUS DIVINE HEALING CAN BE PRODUCED.[36]

Roberts started his ministry in the Bible Belt areas of the Southern States, but his main contribution to modern Christianity was his innovative use of the media – first radio and later television – as a tool of evangelism. In 1956, the *American Magazine* proclaimed him the 'King of the Faith Healers' and by 1969 his programmes were attracting vast audiences across the United States and his television 'specials' were receiving critical acclaim for their artistic presentation. His 'Roberts Valentine Special' received Emmy nominations in 1971 in the categories of art direction, scenic design and lighting direction. More importantly, he was reaching people who no longer attended church and had established the prototype for the modern electronic church. By the end of 1972, his specials were being presented by over 400 stations and his showcase stars included Jimmy Durante, Jerry Lewis, Johnny Mathis, Pearl Bailey and Burl Ives. This parade of Hollywood talent was supplemented by numerous politicians who welcomed Roberts to their districts for on-location productions, and his format of combining religion with entertainment was soon adopted by many imitators. Inevitably, this development became entangled with the realm of big business and some TV evangelists have been severely criticized for the claims they have made, or implied, such as, 'If you get up and touch the TV set you will be healed.' Others are known to have faked miraculous healings on live TV,[37] while the financial and sexual scandals associated with some TV evangelists are now common knowledge. Viewers should always be aware of these negative aspects of commercial evangelism when they watch such programmes.

Like most TV evangelists, Oral Roberts endorsed the Faith Confession Movement. Also known as Prosperity Evangelism, this is based on the idea that spiritual laws exist which, like the laws of physics, are immutable and universal. One such law is that any financial contribution made to God's work that exceeds tithing and prudent giving always brings a generous reward on the investment. Roberts speaks of this as the Miracle of Seed Faith and he discusses the implications in his book of that title, a book that has attracted a wide readership and sold more than two million copies.[38] Put simply, it expounds the idea that God expects his children to prosper financially as well as spiritually.

It was possibly his belief in God's providence that encouraged Roberts to undertake the most spectacular venture of his healing ministry, a project that was to cost $150 million. This was the Roberts' City of Faith, Medical and Research Center, which he opened in 1978. It was located in Tulsa near his university, and Roberts predicted that by 1988 the Center would be regarded as the Mayo Clinic of the Southwest. The complex included graduate schools in medicine, dentistry and nursing, a thirty-storey hospital and facilities for research into cancer, ageing and heart disease. Each patient was assigned a nurse, a physician and a prayer partner, a requirement that reflected Roberts' belief in the importance of a holistic approach to healing.[39] Unfortunately, his venture was overcome by severe financial problems and the project was never completed. The Center closed in 1989.[40]

Whilst creating these facilities for the sick, Roberts also expected people to accept responsibility for their own health. In his book *Your Road to Recovery* he asks:

How much health do you want to have?

Are you willing to quit smoking or give up other bad health habits in order to get God's best health for you?

He encouraged patients to live sensible lives and accept the treatment provided by conventional medicine, and taught that a person can be healed by God and yet remain troubled because they do not follow proper healthcare practices. He wrote many articles and books, and gave this advice to those seeking healing.[41]

> Look on Jesus as a lifesaver, delighting to bless and heal you. Believe that God's abundance of life is for you and you may have it by believing. Know that God's will is to heal not only others, but you. Healing is in the atonement therefore it includes all. Remember that healing begins within – you reach God and He reaches you through your soul. Know that the only way you can overcome your fear is through your faith in God. Use a point of contact through your release of faith. Close the case out for Victory. Join yourself to companions of faith.

From the psychological perspective this is very good advice. The tone is positive and life-affirming. Roberts points to the need to deal with one's inner problems and tells us the best way of doing so. The suggestions are firmly based in the Christian tradition, stressing the importance of first looking to Jesus and his redemption; and then encouraging those in need to reach up to God, or to use the words of the Latin mass, *sursum cordae*, 'lift up your hearts'. What he meant by 'a point of contact' can be interpreted in various ways. The most obvious way to make contact is through the sacraments – the Eucharist or Holy Communion Service – and by prayer, and for this purpose quiet repetitive prayer is particularly useful.

Agnes Sanford found the Jesus Prayer most helpful, and a rapidly increasing number of Christians now follow the lead of the Benedictine monk, John Main, and use a mantra. Some people may consider this practice as being too close to Eastern forms of worship, but the quiet repetition of a short prayer, was recommended by the fourth-century monk Cassian, who was born in Romania and lived in Bethlehem and Egypt. Any short prayer is effective, though John Main favoured the use of 'Marana tha', the Aramaic words meaning 'Come, O Lord' with which St Paul concluded the First Letter to the Corinthians.

Chapter Seven
Other Famous Healers

When I retired, I became a guide at Coventry Cathedral and for almost ten years have enjoyed meeting visitors from many parts of the world and explaining the significance of the building to them. Most are Christians, but I meet Jews, Muslims, Sikhs, atheists and people who are uncertain of what they believe all converging, in a sense as pilgrims, on that spot. I like to emphasize the important contributions made by women and refugees from the Holocaust to the construction of the cathedral and will usually take visitors into the Chapel of Unity, which provides a focal point where Christians of different traditions can draw closer together. The idea of building such a chapel was first mooted in the 1940s, soon after the old cathedral was destroyed by fire bombs, and it was a visionary idea in those days when Christianity was very divided and churches tended to be wary of one another. It would have been difficult to imagine then that the new cathedral would have a special chapel where the Catholic mass would be celebrated each Thursday, and a German Lutheran service held once a fortnight. I welcome the fact that barriers between the mainstream Christian churches are being broken down and see the need for the spirit of acceptance to be extended to other faiths, particularly those with close historical links to Christianity.

In this respect there is a striking difference between the practice of medicine and religion in general. The former is usually open to new ideas and eager to learn from other disciplines; the latter has always had to be exclusive in order to retain the integrity of the faith. Such an approach fuels antipathy towards other religions and is evident in the rejection of anything suggestive of spiritualism that is a feature of Christian and Jewish doctrine. The roots of this antagonism can be found in the ancient biblical attitude to witches and the subsequent belief that all their works are of the devil, even when they seem to be beneficial. I reject entirely the concept, still held in certain circles, that 'healing can be of the Devil'. Wholeness is the gift of God and those who deliver it must be His agents whatever their religious persuasion or outward appearances may be. So far we have concentrated on Christian healers, those who look to Christ as the ultimate source of their healing power. Most heal-ers, however, do not belong to this tradition and yet have a long and rewarding ministry to the sick. Their healing role needs to be considered.

National Federation of Spiritual Healers

Some of the best known healers are Spiritualists – people belonging to a Spiritualist Church or holding similar beliefs. A 'giant' among these was Harry Edwards. He was for many years a successful medium and healer and was also the moving force behind the establishment in 1955 of the National Federation of Spiritual Healers (NFSH). This is an international organization of healers from a wide variety of ethnic, religious and occu-pational backgrounds, including doctors and nurses. In 1987 the NFSH joined with fourteen independent charities to form the Confederation of Healing Organizations (CHO), an umbrella organization which negotiates with government departments and other authoritative bodies on behalf of its members. These include:

- The British Alliance of Healing Organizations
- The College of Psychic Studies
- The Greater World Christian Spiritualist Association
- The Spiritualists' National Union
- The White Eagle Lodge

The Doctor-Healer Network also has a link with the CHO as its chairman is a co-opted member of the CHO committee. These independent groups work closely together to enhance the status of healing. They all provide accredited courses in healing and self-growth, and have the common aim of seeking to ensure that:

> The role and importance of spiritual and lay healing is properly understood, to help healers achieve the highest standards of competence and perform-ance and to establish healing as a standard therapy on the NHS and in pri-vate medicine.[1]

In 1989, the CHO published its Code of Conduct. This includes the requirement that:

1. Its members are insured with the CHO. This is a comprehensive insur-ance that permits the medical profession to prescribe healing or to co-operate with healers without incurring any liability for the conse-quence of healing or of a healer's act.
2. Healers must disclaim an ability to cure, but offer an attempt to heal in some measure.

3. The aim of healers within the CHO membership is to offer a service to the medical profession and to the sick which is a complement and not an alternative to orthodox medicine.
4. Healers should only heal in a conscious state of attunement. Trance conditions are neither recognized in law nor covered by CHO's insurance.
5. Healers must keep adequate records for all patients and ensure that these are kept confidential.[2]

Spiritualism

Most members of the Christian clergy are suspicious of Spiritualists. In their minds they link them with occult practices, such as the use of Tarot cards and Ouija boards, of 'calling up the dead' in darkened rooms, and of healing through 'dark' practices. I remember saying at a Christian healing centre that 'all healing comes from God' and was immediately told by the retreat leader that I was wrong and that healing sometimes comes from the Devil, mentioning spiritualist healing as a specific example. I was so surprised that I failed to remind her that Jesus was accused of healing through 'Beelzebub, prince of devils'[3] and that he replied to this accusation most robustly.

In my experience there is an increasing tendency for people attending Christian healing services to be told that they are devil-possessed and that this is the result of their having attended a Spiritualist church or healer. I find it quite wrong that vulnerable people should be treated in this way. Most Christian clergy in the UK today would be very hesitant to make such derogatory remarks about other major religious faiths such as Islam and Judaism, though vilifying them was often fair game in the past. So to clarify misconceptions, some account needs to be given of what happens in a Spiritualist church.

Healing in Spiritualist Churches

Spiritualism is no longer an outlawed sect. It is an officially recognized religious movement with its own churches and ministers. Spiritualists who need in-patient care have the right to be visited by their ministers and to receive spiritual healing on the wards just like members of other faiths. The fundamental principles of Spiritualism are:

- The Fatherhood of God
- The Brotherhood of Man
- The Communion of Spirits and the Ministry of Angels

- The Continuous Existence of the Human Soul
- Personal responsibility
- Compensation and retribution hereafter for all the good and evil deeds done on earth
- Eternal progress open to every soul.[4]

Members of the Greater World Christian Spiritualist Association also recognize 'the leadership and redemptive power of Jesus Christ'.

Spiritualists do not play about with Ouija boards or table rapping, they do not 'call up the dead' – which they cannot do anyway. Their churches are bright and well lit and the meetings cheerful and relaxed. There are several different types of service each week. The three most common ones are the divine service, the open circle and the healing service. The divine service is held on a Sunday evening and resembles a nonconformist chapel service, with hymns, prayers and a homily; there is also a demonstration of mediumship by a guest medium. It is not an intellectually demanding experience, being much more light-hearted than a church/chapel service with the congregation playing a more active role.

Its distinguishing feature is the presence of the medium. Trance mediums are now a rarity; most mediums work in clear consciousness, standing in front of their audience, chatting to them, answering questions and passing on the messages that they believe they have received from the spirit world. A useful analogy is to see the medium as a teacher standing in front of a group of alert, responsive pupils with whom she/he interacts.

Spiritualism lays great stress on the importance of healing the sick and has done so throughout the twentieth century. There are two approaches to this ministry: personal contact, or 'the laying-on of hands'; and 'absent healing', when healing thoughts and prayers are sent to those in need. Services for the sick are very relaxed. There is no mumbo-jumbo, people walk in and out as they wish, sit down, talk quietly to the healer, receive the healing and then leave. Patients can expect to receive more individual time from the healer than they would at a church service or from their family doctor. There is no charge and no pressure to donate to church funds. Faith is not a requirement and healers claim no special powers, regarding themselves merely as channels conveying energy from the Divine Source to the patient. They see themselves simply as passive agents, have no control over that energy and are unable to direct or influence its natural course in any way. No effort is made to gain converts to Spiritualism.

Not all Christian clergy are prejudiced against Spiritualists. Some are willing to learn. Perhaps typical of them is the priest who wrote the following letter in *Healing Today*:

> As an Anglican priest and a probationer member of the NFSH I have a natural interest in the recent Church report on healing, mentioned in your July

issue. One implication of the report is that, if barriers are to be broken down, there is an impelling need for an informed Christian understanding of the healing movement.[5]

Harry Edwards (1893–1976)

The greatest healer the world has seen since the time of Christ.
Maurice Barbanell [6]

Harry Edwards was a practising Spiritualist and healer. He was born in London where his father was a compositor and his mother, before her marriage, a court dressmaker. She was the undisputed boss of the household and though her children were generally happy and well behaved she dealt quickly with any nonsense. Harry was a troublesome lad, who often had to be corrected, until at the age of twelve he fell for a young girl, Dolly Read, then his conduct changed abruptly. He joined the Church Lads Brigade and persuaded the rest of his gang to stop swearing and behave decently. When Lord Baden-Powell set up the Boy Scouts in 1908, Harry formed one of the first patrols of the movement with a group of ten boys at St Mark's Church, Wood Green. That same year, at the age of fifteen, he became aware of the inequalities in society and joined the Liberal Party, then a major force in British politics.

Harry left school at the age of fourteen and was apprenticed to a printer. He did not enjoy the work but he grafted at it and completed his apprenticeship in 1914. That same year, at the outbreak of the First World War, he volunteered for military service and was posted to India in 1915. He had not been long in that country when he and the padre published an article in the battalion magazine denouncing the attitude of the residents of Bangalore to British soldiers. The soldiers were not allowed to use the public library or certain restaurants, and were banned from the public park where there was a notice stating: 'Dogs and soldiers are not admitted.' The military authorities regarded the article as seditious and court martialled Private Edwards and his co-author. At the trial, Edwards elected to defend himself, but the case was eventually dropped.

In spite of this initial setback, Harry was promoted lance-corporal and posted to the North-West Frontier. There, most remarkably, he was commissioned in the field and sent to Tikrit with instructions to supervise the construction of a railway line between Tikrit and Baghdad. Subsequently he was promoted acting major and posted to north Persia as 'Assistant Director of Labour, Persian Lines of Communication' and given the task of building roads and bridges capable of carrying heavy military equipment. He recruited his work force from local villagers, and they expected him to provide medical care for themselves and their families. He was so success-ful in this role that they called him hakim or doctor, and people came from all parts of the country for treatment. He had no special medical supplies or specialized training, and the treatment he offered was based mainly on common sense and a caring attitude, but it was appreciated.

Although the war ended in 1918 Harry was not discharged from the army until 1921. When he returned to the UK, it was as a staff officer with the rank of major, a remarkable achievement for someone who had left school at the age of fourteen. He then set up his own printing business, married, started a family and renewed his interest in politics. He rejoined the Liberal Party, now past its heyday, and although he had political ambi-tions and was a parliamentary candidate on several occasions, he was never elected to Parliament. During this time he was also an active worker for the League of Nations.

Harry was brought up in the Church of England but became a regular attender of the Spiritualist Church following the death of his nephew, Nigel, in a road traffic accident in 1936. He was greatly impressed by the standard of the communications given at these meetings, both to himself and to members of his family, and he eventually became a practising medium him-self. He also developed an interest in healing. This is not surprising as 'healing' has been an integral part of this Church's ministry since the nine-teenth century and members are encouraged and trained to be healers.

The first person Harry cured by 'hands-on healing' was Gladys Cudd, a young girl with tuberculosis. She was so ill that her parents had spread straw on the road outside the house to quieten the noise of passing traffic. When Harry visited her, she was already unconscious and wanting to help, but not knowing what to do, he placed his hands gently on her head and asked for her to be healed. Suddenly, he became aware of a strange sensa-tion. He felt that he was being rooted to the floor and that his body was being filled with an energy that flowed through his arms and hands into Gladys. There was no shaking or quivering, just a flow of energy, which slowly diminished and then ceased. He was filled with an exalted feeling of joy and confidence. Gladys's recovery was not instantaneous, but it was swift and complete.[7]

At the outbreak of the Second World War, Harry was 46 years old, too old for military service. During the war, he worked as a printer by day and as a healer by night: he also joined the Home Guard. In 1944, his home was bombed and all the records of his patients were destroyed. This was most disheartening and when he spoke of it later he said:

> It was as if the very bottom had fallen out of life itself, for I knew that the Absent Healing work had received a very heavy blow. All I could then do was record from memory as many cases as I could for direct intercession and conduct a mass intercession for the remainder.[8]

Harry received no payment for the absent healing work.

In 1946, he decided to concentrate all his energies on healing. He gave his printing business to his brother, bought a large country house, called Burrows Lea, in Surrey, and established a healing sanctuary there. He now had enough space to employ a small band of secretaries to help with the hundreds of letters that arrived each week requesting absent healing and other forms of help. In this work he was assisted by Olive and George Burton, and later by Ray and Joan Branch, who still maintain a healing ministry at Burrows Lea. They also continue to publish the journal *The Spiritual Healer*, which Harry started and which is sent free of charge to interested readers.

Whilst many people were willing to help him with his healing ministry, Harry always said that his main support came from his spirit guides. He was convinced that he was being used as a healing channel by discarnate spirits, and in particular by the spirits of Louis Pasteur, the French microbiologist, and Lord Lister, who introduced the practice of antiseptic surgery. He also spoke of a vision that had great significance for him. It occurred whilst he was seated alone in his sanctuary, of it he said:

> there suddenly appeared before me a white-robed, patriarchal figure whose personality conveyed a radiance, tremendously loving, yet commanding in purpose.

The apparition did not speak, but held in his hands a large metal ring, upon which swung three keys. Harry never experienced anything like this again but it left him with a sense of elation and the belief that he was meant to work in partnership with others.[9]

Harry worked very effectively in the peaceful atmosphere of Burrows Lea, but he made his greatest impact in more public arenas. His presence guaranteed a large audience and he gave a most remarkable demonstration of healing in the Royal Albert Hall on 25 September 1954. This was the first big meeting organized by the newly-formed National Federation of Spiritual Healers, which Harry had helped to establish and which elected him as its first president.[10] Those present at the Royal Albert Hall included representatives from the British Medical Association and from the Church's Council of Healing, as well as seventeen members of a Commission on Divine Healing which had been set up by the Archbishops of Canterbury and York.

Harry was also a trance medium; this aspect of his life's work is easily overlooked as his healing was always done in clear consciousness. He did not exercise this gift in public but on Monday evenings he would sit with close colleagues and go into a trance, and then review the week's work with the aid of a spirit guide, called Reuben. These sessions, which would last about an hour, were taped so that a permanent record was available of the discussions that Reuben had with the group each week. Anything relating to healing might be brought up at these seminars.

Harry was also a prolific writer though he typed with only one finger and published many articles and books on healing.[11] He did not have unqualified success as a healer, nor was his optimism always well founded. He tried to help my cousin, Rhoyd, who had Pott's disease (tuberculosis of the spine) before the advent of anti-TB drugs. Rhoyd was then a teenager and he persuaded his mother to take him to Harry for treatment. Rhoyd came away convinced that he would be cured, but the treatment was ineffective and his back became deformed.

Rhoyd's subsequent disappointment underlined for me the importance of not creating unrealistic expectations or making promises that cannot be kept. Healers should never exaggerate their capabilities, and members of the NFSH do not do so, but when I was a hospice doctor we were involved with a family who sought help from a Sikh healer for their teenage son who was dying of cancer. She reassured them that he would be cured and rarely have I seen such distress and despair in a family when he died a few weeks later.

George Chapman (1921–)

George Chapman was another Spiritualist healer of international repute. I first heard about him from a Catholic priest, Fr Kenneth Gillespie, a family friend and Franciscan friar, who served a parish in mid-Wales. One day he told me that he had just visited a lady who had been healed of cancer by a discarnate doctor and that I should visit her. The lady was Elma Williams, a writer of animal books who lived with a motley collection of livestock at Pant Glas, a homestead in a remote Welsh valley.

Fr Gillespie kept referring to Elma's recovery whenever I met him and eventually, when my wife and children were away, I phoned Ms Williams and asked if I might visit her and have a chat. Her immediate reply was no, adding that the place was in a dreadful mess: but when in response I mentioned that I had just been feeding the children's horses, she relented and invited me along. I found Pant Glas in a narrow valley containing just this one house and numerous horses, donkeys, sheep, goats, domestic pets and poultry, including a golden cockerel called Augustus who wandered in and out of the house as if he owned the place.

We talked at length and she spoke of being crippled by secondary bone cancer and of constant pain, until a friend suggested that she should visit George Chapman, a healer in Aylesbury. She wrote, but could not get an appointment for at least six months, so her friend gave up his place and, with considerable difficulty, she went to Aylesbury just three weeks later, where she met George Chapman and his spirit guide, Dr William Lang.

The consultation was a success and she continued to receive absent healing. When I saw her two years later she was pain-free and mobile, though
her movements were restricted by stiffness in the back. If I remember rightly, the primary site of the cancer was in the breast.

George Chapman left school when he was fourteen. During the Second
World War, he served in the Royal Air Force reaching the rank of sergeant.
He was demobilized in 1946 when he joined the Aylesbury Fire Brigade.
One of the firemen at the station was interested in Spiritualism, a subject
new to Chapman. He wanted to learn more about it so attended a
Spiritualist church and was so impressed with what he heard that he spent
time trying to develop his own psychic abilities. Some months later, and
quite inadvertently, he realized that he possessed the gift of healing. By this
time he had also mastered the art of entering a deep trance with ease. His
biographer, Bernard Hutton,[12] who was himself cured of blindness by
Chapman/Dr Lang, says that during these trances George was being
specifically trained to be the medium for Dr Lang, a former ophthalmic
surgeon.

This association became a working reality in 1951 and from that date the
two worked together as a team. People would come to George with their
complaints, he would go into a trance and allow the discarnate Dr Lang to
possess his body and heal the patient. It may seem a bizarre arrangement
but this is the way it worked and eventually people travelled from all over
the world to consult Dr Lang. The Canadian artist Lucille Gilling reveals in
her book *Bright Shines the Sunlight* how her vision was much improved by
the treatment given by Dr Lang, and quotes the following testimony by
Marie Lyndon Lang, Dr Lang's daughter:

> the person who speaks through George Chapman and claims to be William
> Lang is without doubt my father . . .We asked many questions of father about
> things only he could know. He knew all the answers and better still he could
> ask questions in return.[13]

My interest in George Chapman was rekindled about twenty years after
I had met Elma Williams when a Macmillan nurse asked me to visit a terminally ill patient in Birmingham. The man, who was dying from lung
cancer, told us that he had just been to see George Chapman, that George
now lived at Pant Glas and that he was hoping to see him again soon.
Apparently, when Elma Williams died, George bought Pant Glas, possibly
because it was on a ley line with Glastonbury, a focal point of early British
Christianity and centre of spiritual energy. He was now a full-time professional healer holding clinics in Pant Glas and in France. Our patient was
too ill to travel far and never returned to consult George again, but his family, knowing of my interest, asked George if I might visit him. The response
was positive and some years later, after I had retired, I went to Pant Glas

and we had a long session together which was a most generous gesture on his part.

My first impression was that the valley had changed completely. The grounds were tidier and a special healing clinic had been built close to the house, which had itself been renovated. George's son welcomed me and took me into the clinic to meet his father. After the preliminary courtesies George went into a trance and I met Dr Lang.

The historical Dr William Lang was a prominent ophthalmic surgeon, who worked in London between 1875 and 1930. Various people who knew him in life, including his daughter and granddaughter,[14] have affirmed that the person speaking through George Chapman is this surgeon but the available facts are obviously open to different interpretations. William Lang was born in Exeter in 1852, the son of a Moravian merchant. He was educated at Lausanne and at the London Hospital, where he registered as a medical student in 1870 and qualified in 1874. His wife and childhood sweetheart, Emma, died in 1892. He became a Fellow of the Royal College of Surgeons (FRCS) in 1879, ophthalmic surgeon to the Middlesex Hospital in 1880 and consultant surgeon to the Central London Ophthalmic Hospital (now Moorfields Eye Hospital) in 1884. He was a leading ophthalmic surgeon in the first two decades of the twentieth century, published original research work in medical journals, and was President of the Ophthalmological Section of the Royal Society of Medicine. He died in July 1937 holding the book *The Life of Jesus*, by Ernest Renan, in his hands.[15]

The 'person' I met through George Chapman was a courteous, elderly gentleman who addressed me as 'young man' in a brisk authoritative way. The transition from medium to elderly doctor was almost instantaneous, and in appearance and voice the two were entirely different. As Dr Lang, George Chapman's body seemed to shrink, his face appeared thinner and more elderly, and the voice slightly higher pitched and clearer. I have almost no recollection of what was said, but for the most part Dr Lang did the speaking whilst I listened. However, when George and I spoke privately later, the conversation was more evenly balanced.

I did not seek healing from Dr Lang and cannot give a firsthand account of the way in which his treatment is carried out, but this has been well documented by others.[16] Apparently, Dr Lang works with spirit assistants, including his son Basil, who was himself a qualified doctor. There may be some passage of the hands over the clothed body to facilitate the diagnosis and then during the healing procedure, which is conducted like a surgical operation, the patient is aware of instructions being given to assistants and of the snapping of fingers as spirit instruments are used and discarded. The discarnate team work quickly and the psychic operation is completed in a few minutes. The healing provided is supplemented by continued distant healing.

Edgar Cayce (1877–1945)

A seer out of season.
Harmon H. Bro

Edgar Cayce was not a healer in the generally accepted sense of the term. He did not pray for people or lay his hands on them, but twice a day he would lie down and go into a prayerful trance. In that state he would consider the problems that people brought to his attention by means of telephone calls or through the mail, and then dictate to his secretary the advice to be given in each case. During these sessions, his wife, Gertrude, would sit nearby to support him and, towards the end of the reading, would ask questions to clarify the instructions he had given.[17] The sitting would last about an hour and was a regular procedure over many years.

Born on a farm in Kentucky, Edgar Cayce learnt at an early age to look after animals, sow and harvest crops, cure tobacco, preserve fruit and vegetables and generally be useful about the homestead. He fished in the stream, hunted quail, rode horses bareback and developed a close affinity with the natural world. His father was a justice of the peace, but the young lad especially enjoyed the company of his grandparents, particularly his grandfather, who took him fishing and told him stories of his encounters with those who had recently died. Tragically, his grandfather died after being trampled by a horse. Cayce was devastated and he only came to terms with his loss when, some months later, he had a strong sense that his grandfather was still a living presence.[18]

Cayce was a studious lad who had read the Bible twelve times before he was thirteen years old. He enjoyed church activities, became an elder of his church and was a Sunday school teacher for many years. In 1889, when he was twelve, he was baptized by total immersion: that night he had a vision, in which a figure appeared to him in a radiant light and told him that 'his prayers had been heard: he would have his wish: he was to remain faithful: to be true to himself: and that he was to help the sick and afflicted'. He slept little that night and was in such a daze the next day that he could not spell simple words when tested at school. The teacher was his uncle and he reported this to Edgar's father who decided to give his son extra tuition in spelling. The boy made many mistakes and was punished with frequent cuffs to the head until his father went to the kitchen for a drink, then Edgar rested his head on the book, prayed and dozed for a few moments. When his father returned Edgar could spell all the words in the book and later he was able to memorize passages from any book using the same technique. This new facility lasted for the rest of his life.[19]

Two years later, he received another severe blow to the head, this time whilst playing a ball game at school. He was so disoriented that his sister took him home where he was put to bed and fell into a deep sleep. While still asleep he began to speak clearly and authoritatively, giving instructions on the treatment that was needed to prevent brain damage. Then he commented on a number of issues that would be helpful to his parents.

Later, his father admitted that he would have benefited financially if he had followed his son's advice, though it must also be noted that Cayce's own financial adventures in later life tended to be unsuccessful. These included the establishment at Virginia Beach, in 1928, of a 'psychic' hospital, where practitioners diagnosed patients' complaints by psychic concentration. The first physician appointed to the centre was Dr House. He had a longstanding acquaintance with Cayce's methods, and was qualified in medicine and osteopathy. He died in 1929 aged fifty-two, and was replaced by Dr Lydic, an osteopath. The hospital was well endowed, receiving over $100,000 from business associates of Edgar Cayce but, perhaps as a consequence of the 1929 Wall Street crash, it was forced to close in 1931.

Cayce left school at the age of sixteen and worked first as a shop assistant, then as a travelling salesman and photographer. At the age of thirty-three, now a married man and father, he became a 'psychic diagnostician' in partnership with a Mr Noe and a Dr Ketchum. The following year his second child died in infancy and his wife developed tuberculosis. Her condition deteriorated so rapidly that the attending physician, Dr Jackson, took Cayce aside and said, 'if there's anything in this monkey business you've been doing with these fellows around here, you better try it on your wife.'[20] Dr Jackson expected Gertrude to die within the week and in his account of this period Cayce wrote:

> Will anyone ever understand what it meant to me to know that I was taking the life of one near and dear to me in my own hands, and that the very forces and powers that I had been so wishy-washy in using for years must now be put to the crucial test.[21]

He went into a trance and recommended a prescription which the pharmacist had never previously dispensed, but when the medicine was given to his wife, the haemorrhages stopped and she began to recover. He also said that she should inhale the fumes of apple brandy from a charred oak keg. The illness brought Edgar and Gertrude closer together and she became more involved in his work with the sick. He now severed his connection with Ketchum and Noe.

Cayce was a deeply religious man with a firm belief in reincarnation as was sometimes apparent in the trance readings he provided. He was psychically gifted and firmly rejected the suggestion that he acted as a medium, insisting that he followed a procedure that enabled him to access the information he required by using a combination of clairvoyance and religious guidance. The readings were meticulously filed, particularly in his later years, and these files eventually contained details of the advice given to the approximately 9,000 people who had sought his help.[22] Requests for help came from all over the United States, usually by mail, but the letters were often supplemented by telephone calls and telegrams. The requests were so numerous that he never needed to advertise and, apart from one short period, never did so.

When he came out of trance Cayce was never aware of what he had said during it, but the recommendations were always holistically based and he invariably remembered those who had contacted him previously. There was a pattern to much of the advice he gave. He told everyone to drink six to eight glasses of water a day and his advocacy of high colonic irrigations was almost a Cayce trademark. The files also reveal that he frequently suggested the application of hot flannel packs containing castor oil, fasting and special diets. Cayce was not fiercely ascetic, more Epicurean: he approved of a moderate approach to the good things of life, and advised against excessive anxiety and uncertainty, encouraging people to take full responsibility for their own lives and not to allow the inner cancer of dislike and distrust become a virulent malignant growth.

He was keenly aware of the need for spiritual development and said that this often entailed personal discipline with God-centredness taking the place of self-centredness. This did not require martyrdom but the setting aside of those preoccupations which were no longer meaningful and which needed to be discarded. He also believed that people should sometimes accept hardships so that they could understand what others were enduring, and thereby become filled with the desire to help. He used to say that the inner prayer of Jesus, which enabled him to be faithful to the Cross, was 'Others, Lord. Others.'[23]

Dr Mikao Usui (?–1926)

Founder of Reiki.

Some healers are notable not so much for their personal ministry as for the healing systems they formulated. Dr Usui, the founder of *Reiki* (pronounced Ray Key), was one such person. *Reiki* is a Japanese word meaning 'universal life energy', but the term is also used for the method of hands-on healing that Dr Usui devised and which is now practised by many therapists throughout the world. Surprisingly little is known about Dr Usui, especially of his early life. Few written records are available and there is some uncertainty about the authenticity of the stories that have been told about him, but some facts are irrefutable.

Dr Mikao Usui acquired his healing skills in Japan, probably towards the end of the nineteenth century. It is also likely that he shared the traditional beliefs prevalent in Japan at that time, accepting the reality of the *kami*, the ancestral spirits, who, among their other attributes, retain a close interest in our world of human affairs.

We are told that Dr Usui was the president of Doshisha University, a small Christian foundation in Kyoto, where he was also a Christian minister. One Sunday morning, a senior student asked him whether he accepted the contents of the Bible literally, he replied 'yes'. The student then asked if he believed in the healing miracles recorded in the Bible, and to this he also answered 'yes', qualifying the reply by saying that he had however never witnessed a healing. The student went on to suggest that 'blind faith' was sufficient for an old person like Dr Usui, but not enough for students at the beginning of their careers. This exchange made a great impression on him, and the next day Dr Usui resigned his position as president of Doshisha University and left for the United States.[24]

In the United States he attended Chicago University where he obtained his doctorate in Christian doctrine, but in spite of all this learning he was still unable to heal in the way that Jesus and his disciples had done. Eventually, he returned to Japan where he visited Buddhist monasteries, studied the scriptures and talked to Buddhist monks. But they were not helpful, considering themselves to be too busy with people's spiritual problems to have any time for their physical suffering.

He continued his search for seven years. During this time he read manuscripts in various languages, including Chinese and Sanskrit. Eventually he chanced upon a document, written by an unknown monk, containing verbatim statements attributed to the Buddha. It described the healing techniques used by the Buddha and the symbols he employed: this gave Dr Usui the theoretical knowledge he required, but he still lacked the power to heal. He discussed his problem with a friendly abbot, and following this meeting went to one of the sacred mountains of Japan to be alone and to meditate on the significance of the symbols. He was there for twenty-one days. On the first day he placed twenty-one stones in front of him, and as each day passed he cast a stone away.

On the last day, he still had not achieved his goal but, as he sat meditating, a great ball of light rushed towards him and struck him. Then in rapid succession he saw each symbol like a bubble of light before him. He awoke from the trance refreshed and strengthened, and started his descent of the mountain. As he walked he stumbled and stubbed a toe. His natural reaction was to hold it and as he did so the pain went away and the bleeding ceased. Further down the hillside, he stopped to buy food at a booth. The food was brought to him by the owner's daughter who was suffering from toothache. With her parents' permission, he touched her face and the pain and swelling subsided. On reaching the monastery, he learnt that his friend the abbot was in bed with acute arthritis. After washing and eating, Dr Usui visited the abbot, placed his hands on him and relieved his pain.

For the next seven years he worked amongst the poor, healing their physical ailments, but he could not help noticing that this did not help them to escape from their poverty, or even to show much desire to do so. This saddened him because he believed that physical healing is not sufficient in itself. He then set out the *Five Precepts of Reiki* to help people regulate their inner lives and harmonize their thoughts. These precepts are:

- Just for today do not anger.
- Just for today do not worry.
- Earn your living honestly.
- Honour your parents, elders and teachers.
- Give gratitude to every living thing and every situation.[25]

Reiki is one of the fastest-growing therapies in the world. It is a touch therapy used by those who have learnt the method and then been initiated into the *Reiki* system at a simple but sacred ceremony. The first person to be trained by Dr Usui was a retired naval officer, Chujiro Hayashi. He established a clinic in Tokyo where he taught *Reiki* healing to Hawayo Takata, a young woman from Hawaii. She took the technique to the Americas and the treatment is now widely available. A healing session lasts about 45–60 minutes, during which time patients lie comfortably on a couch. They do not need to undress, but it is best to loosen tight clothing to facilitate relaxation. The therapist heals by resting his/her hands gently on the body, starting with the eyes and moving around the head and down the trunk. By this simple procedure the 'universal life force' is transmitted to the patient. The therapist does not have to seek attunement with the spirit world or with their God before acting as a healing conduit.

Sai Baba (1926–)

Sai Baba is not a Christian or a Spiritualist. He is a Hindu guru who is regarded by his followers as an avatar, an incarnate god, and he is probably one of the most influential spiritual teachers in India today. Like other well-known gurus, his influence extends beyond the Indian subcontinent and his followers are found in many different countries.[26] They include the mentally deranged and depressed and, in August 2001, *The Times*[27] reported the death of three young Britons who committed suicide following visits to Sai Baba centres. Despite these tragedies, I think it worth describing one of his healings because it underlines the fact that no one culture has a monopoly of miraculous cures.

I became interested in Sai Baba when I read a brief report in the *British Medical Journal* describing the successful treatment of a man with severe, spasmodic torticollis (muscle spasm of the neck).[28] I knew how intractable the problem can be for I was involved with such a patient when I worked in a psychiatric unit in South Wales in 1960. The patient, a man aged about forty, had been placed in my care when I joined the hospital staff as a Senior House Officer. He had already consulted many specialists – physicians, surgeons and psychiatrists – who had been unable to help him in any way, and I soon realized that something extraordinary, a minor miracle perhaps, would be needed to bring him relief. I never achieved any improvement in his condition so I was fascinated to learn of someone who had cured a similar disability.

Sai Baba's given name was Sathyanarayana Raju. He was born in a village in South India and brought up in a pious family. In his youth he used to organize prayer meetings for the other children and compose religious songs. He was a good poet, singer and dancer, enjoyed sports and was a keen member of the Boy Scouts. It is reported that sometimes he would go into ecstatic trances and materialize gifts for his friends, which annoyed his father and caused angry confrontations between them. On one occasion, when he was about fourteen years old, his father was so angry that he exploded with the question 'Are you a god, or a ghost, or a madcap? Tell me.' The boy replied, 'I am Sai Baba', implying that he was the reincarnation of a local saint. Soon afterwards he left the village, but returned some years later to establish an ashram for his followers. He used to say that his life had three distinct phases: the first sixteen years were devoted to sports, the next sixteen were characterized by miraculous events, and the last phase would be remembered for his teaching.[29] Some of his followers see him primarily as a notable healer, but he considers that his main work in life is the teaching of spiritual truths.

Sai Baba's healing of the man with torticollis was reported in the *British Medical Journal* by a consultant neurologist then working in the Middle East. He himself had failed to cure the man, as had other doctors and healers. A few weeks after consulting the neurologist, the man returned with no obvious disability, this time selling life insurance policies. He explained that following their previous meeting he had gone to Sai Baba's ashram where he had sat in utter despondency. Then Sai Baba walked by, placed a hand on his head and said that with God's blessing his worries would soon be over. He spent a week at the ashram where he rapidly improved and returned home feeling well and normal. According to the neurologist he had been transformed into a happy and smiling individual, completely cured.[30]

F. M. Alexander (1869–1955)

Founder of the Alexander Technique.

F. M. Alexander was not a spiritual healer but he had a clear understanding of the way that poor posture can lead to ill health, and he relieved many people of their disabilities by teaching them to stand and sit properly. Alexander was born in Tasmania. He started his career as a Shakespearean actor but after a few years he found that by the end of each performance his voice was weak and hoarse. He realized that he must find an answer to this problem, so he began to analyse carefully what happened when he was acting and noticed that the muscles at the back of his neck tended to tighten, that his head would collapse back and downwards on to his neck, and that he would appear shorter in stature. He observed other physical changes as well, all of which tended to diminish the strength of his voice. Over a long period of time he learned to correct these tendencies and as his voice improved so did his general sense of well-being; he also became stronger and fitter. From this basis he formulated the Alexander Technique and started to teach it in Sydney, Australia.

The Alexander Technique is based on the premise that the way a person uses their body affects their general health. Strictly speaking it is a 'taught technique' not a 'healing', but its potential to enhance a person's sense of well-being is such that it merits inclusion here. Most major colleges of music and drama throughout the world, including the Royal Academy of Dramatic Art, the Royal College of Music and the Royal Academy of Music, teach the Alexander Technique. It can be regarded as an essential skill for the professional actor and musician and has many health benefits for the ordinary individual.

There are over 1,000 teachers of the Technique world-wide and a three-year full-time training programme is available for those wishing to become teachers.[31] On a first visit the Alexander teacher notes how the client sits, stands and walks and then shows them how to perform these simple acts without strain or discomfort. This is so important, as a GP I was aware that many of the problems I saw in the surgery were due to poor posture when sitting. This fault needed to be corrected, though I found it almost impossible to persuade people to change the way they sat or stood. Alexander teachers are much more successful, possibly because they can devote 30–60 minutes to each patient session and up to thirty visits may be necessary to rectify the problem.

The high incidence of back problems underlines the need for people to be much more health conscious when choosing their household furniture. We should give greater consideration to the effect that sitting on low-lying sofas and chairs can have on our musculo-skeletal systems and of the pain and disability that we may suffer as a result. Manufacturers should also be encouraged to consult experts on posture before deciding on the design of new furniture for the home and office. Much thought should also be given to the seats installed in public and private transport systems. Motorists often spend two hours a day sitting in their vehicles, lorry drivers a lot longer.

Dr Edward Bach (1886–1936)

Deviser of the Bach Flower Remedies.

People all over the world take the flower remedies devised by Dr Bach. His is a household name among those interested in complementary medicine but it is less well known among members of the medical profession even though he himself was a qualified doctor, who worked in some of the most famous London hospitals and practised in Harley Street.

Dr Bach was an English physician of Welsh ancestry. The Welsh word '*bach*' means small or little one, so it is likely that his ancestors tended to be on the short side. He was born in Birmingham and studied medicine in London where he worked as a bacteriologist in University College Hospital. I often wonder if the job suited him as he preferred the open countryside to towns, and a hospital laboratory appointment would have given him few opportunities for direct contact with patients. On the other hand, I am constantly surprised at the relatively large number of spiritually sensitive medical doctors who work in laboratories.

During the First World War, Dr Bach was declared unfit for military service; instead, he undertook a large clinical workload at University College Hospital where he collapsed with rectal bleeding in 1917. Two years later, after major surgery for this condition, he accepted a post at the London Homeopathic Hospital and became interested in the ideas of Samuel Hahnemann, the founder of homeopathy. He also set up in private practice in Harley Street.

It is said that Bach was a natural healer who could cure instantaneously. This may be so but there are not many recorded accounts of such healings, and he seems to have coupled an intuitive understanding of what people needed with a disconcerting frankness. He had his own instinctive ideas about the causes of disease and the way they should be treated, believing that a person's personality and attitude to life should be the main guide when choosing the best remedy, not the disease itself.

Bach was interested in people and would probably have made a good psychiatrist, but he practised at a time when this was a relatively new discipline. He was interested in people's personalities and their emotional problems, and he came to the conclusion that there were seven basic moods that were so debilitating that they were responsible for much illness. These moods were: fear, uncertainty, lack of interest, loneliness, over-sensitivity, despondency or despair, and over-concern for other people's problems. He also believed that nature had provided a herbal remedy for each of these conditions, and the search for these remedies became the great goal of the last few years of his life.

Bach selected twelve plants, which he intuitively decided would relieve his patients of these moods. He called the plants the 'Twelve Healers'. They were the rock rose, mimulus, cerato, scleranthus, gentian, clematis, water violet, impatiens, agrimony, centaury, chicory and vervain. He later chose other plants which he believed would assist the healing process, these he called the 'Seven Helpers'.

Eventually, he formulated the 'Thirty-eight Bach Flower Remedies' to which he added the 'Rescue Remedy' with which, it is reputed, he saved a fisherman's life in 1930. The 'Rescue Remedy' is a blend of five of the original remedies, it is many people's favourite and I know of one GP's wife who gives it to her husband when she thinks he needs a tonic. The remedies can be bought over the counter in health food shops and some people treat their plants and animals with them. The easiest way to treat plants in the garden is to put 5–10 drops of the appropriate remedy in a gallon of water and sprinkle it around with a watering can.

Bach received the core inspiration for his healing system whilst walking in North Wales. He was crossing a field heavy with dew, when he realized that each dew drop contained the essence of the plant on which it lay and that the potency of the essence would be enhanced by the heat of the sun. He concluded that the liquid would have health-giving properties and soon found that adequate quantities of a chosen remedy could be extracted if a few blooms from the relevant plant were placed in a glass of clear, spring water and allowed to stand in full sunlight for several hours. He made infusions of all his remedies in this way and, following homeopathic principles, enhanced their potency by diluting and shaking them. He added alcohol as a preservative and a few drops of each remedy is all the patient, plant or animal requires. Because the active ingredient is not a physical agent but the life force of the plant itself, there is no risk of overdosage.[32]

In his book *The Twelve Healers and Other Remedies*, Dr Bach says that there should be no difficulty in selecting a remedy to effect a cure. He also advises healers to 'Take no notice of the disease, think only of the outlook on life of the one in distress'.[33] His remedies are suitable for people of all ages and more than one can be given simultaneously, the Rescue Remedy is also available as a cream. Dr Bach's approach has inspired others to create their own flower derived medicines.[34] These are usually called 'Flower Essences' to distinguish them from Dr Bach's remedies, and include essences of desert cacti, Australian bush flowers, and the wild flowers of many other countries.

Sir Harold Ridley (1906–2001)

Father of the Modern Cataract Operation.

It is only too easy to overlook the immense contributions that twentieth-century medicine has made to the welfare of people all over the world. Blindness must surely be one of the worst burdens to bear, leading, as it does, to total loss of independence as well as all those pleasures that sight provides. Six million people are relieved of this burden each year as a result of the vision and determination of Harold Ridley. He was not a healer in the conventional sense of the word nor did his become a household name like Dr Bach and Sai Baba. He was an ophthalmic surgeon whose skill turned a dream into a reality.

Harold Ridley was born in Leicestershire where his father was also an ophthalmic surgeon. His mother was a friend of Florence Nightingale and he could recall sitting on her knee as a boy. He qualified as a doctor in 1930, at St Thomas's Hospital, where he was later to perform the landmark operation which eye care professionals rate as one of the great advances in this branch of medicine. It enabled people with cataract to regain almost normal vision without the aid of spectacles.

Pioneering the use of the intraocular lens (IOL) was Ridley's major contribution to eye care, but he helped in other important ways also. In 1941 he was posted, with the Royal Army Medical Corps, to Ghana where he undertook original work in the field of tropical eye disease, identifying river blindness (onchocerciasis), a disease caused by a minute parasite, which is prevalent in certain parts of Africa and South America. On his return to the UK, Ridley was appointed consultant surgeon at St Thomas's Hospital where a student suggested that a lens damaged by cataract, could be replaced by a clear lens. 'Many hundreds of people, including myself, had suggested this project,' Ridley recalled. 'However, no one had the temerity to take action.' Most people thought the operation would be too difficult and that the lens would be rejected by the body's immune system. During the war, however, Ridley had operated on injured airmen to remove fragments of Perspex cockpit canopy that had been embedded in their eyes. He noted that the fragments rarely caused any reaction in the eye, and realized that this substance had the potential to be excellent lens material. He held a series of secret meetings, one in his car, with like-minded specialists, including John Pike an optical scientist, and obtained a sample of Perspex from the manufacturers, ICI.

The first operation was done in two parts. The patient was a 45-year-old woman and her defective lens was removed on 29 November 1949. The new lens was inserted on 8 February 1950. The operation was done in secret as Ridley wanted to avoid all publicity until he was sure that the result could withstand any criticism. Unfortunately, the patient mistakenly went to another Harley Street ophthalmologist, Frederick Ridley, for the follow-up visit and the cover was blown. The leading surgeons of the day were furious. 'Reckless' was the term most often used to describe the innovatory operation. Later Ridley was to say, 'I could not afford a single mistake. The whole world was against it and they were waiting to pounce on me.' Luckily, the good outcome proved the value of the IOL operation. The method was refined and later undertaken as a single procedure. Young doctors now implant IOLs routinely and with ease, not realizing the enormous struggle that Ridley and others had to make to develop this technique.

Cataract surgery with lens implantation is now deemed almost trivial by some, but the comments of a grateful patient, who is also a doctor, may help to summarize the essence of Sir Harold Ridley's legacy. 'Even when a miracle becomes routine' he said, 'it still remains a miracle.'[35] Sir Harold Ridley was very fortunate that his 'miracle' was so clearly demonstrated. There could be no argument about the benefits conferred by his operation. This is not always the case. The claims of other healers are often disputed and any evidence that their ministrations had led to a permanent improvement in their patients' condition is much harder to obtain. It is, however, essential that the search should continue if healing is to be accorded any worthwhile respect.

Chapter Eight
Scientific Studies on Healing

One reason why Western civilization has flourished since the Renaissance has been its commitment to the scientific method, an analytical approach to knowledge in which details are studied, divided and distinguished. This has produced enormous benefits for mankind, but it has had one unfortunate side-effect: the weakening of the link between people and their spiritual roots. In a way it has led to science becoming the new 'god' to which everyone has to make obeisance. Modern science, however, is much more open to spiritual concepts than Newtonian physics was, and since the middle of the twentieth century a spiritual renaissance has swept through the secular world in a remarkable way. This is not due to any efforts by established church leaders – Churches have received their own Baptism of the Spirit, but mainly in Third World countries – the seeds of this revival may be found in the ideas of religious thinkers such as Teilhard de Chardin, Carl Jung and Bede Griffiths. They speak of a new evolution gradually unfolding, this time not of the species but of the human consciousness, which manifests itself in a more mystical approach to life and the search for a spiritual path based on love not dogma. It is perhaps encapsulated in the last lines of Bishop Timothy Rees's hymn, 'God is Love' where he says:

God is Love, so Love for ever
o'er the universe must reign.

or more simply in the Beatles' song:

All you need is love, love,
Love is all you need.

It is possible that researchers are drawn to examine the ministry of the 'healer' in this spirit. Subconsciously they are hoping to prove that love does indeed have the power to transform, and heal, people's lives.

125

Before considering the experiments undertaken to determine the effectiveness of healing, two questions need to be answered: first, can healing be investigated scientifically, and second, should such investigations be undertaken? The answer to the first question is undoubtedly yes. The rigorous examination by the Lourdes Medical Bureau, and its International Medical Committee, of cures claimed by pilgrims to Lourdes, and the introduction of double-blind trials in complementary medicine are just two indications that proper evaluations can be made of claims for healing by unconventional methods.

The answer to the question, 'should such investigations be undertaken?' is more problematic. The Catholic Church has a long history of examining claims made for miraculous cures and believes that such an approach is essential. Others are less certain. Charlatans obviously benefit from a lack of scrutiny and will wish to avoid it, but there is also a body of opinion which believes that any interference in the communication between healer and patient may affect the outcome, comparing the situation to the one found in subatomic physics where the simple act of measurement has an irreversible effect on the activities being studied. The same argument applies, however, to any assessment of medical outcome involving a patient and a healer, including those instances where the healer is a doctor. Here such assessments are commonplace. Moreover, in many countries traditional healers work openly in a public setting and expect their practices to be scrutinized, and do not regard this as limiting their effectiveness in any way, but as an acceptable means of gaining new clients.

Testing Old Methods

It is in the interests of everyone that researchers should test the effectiveness of available remedies. The value of this approach can be shown by considering the different ways that doctors treated three conditions: the strawberry naevus, orf and herpes zoster.

A strawberry naevus is a birthmark. It appears early in infancy as a small red spot, which is usually located on the face or trunk. It grows rapidly and continues to enlarge, acquiring a strawberry-like appearance, until the infant is about eighteen months old. Parents are disturbed by its appearance and growth and are anxious to have it removed. Various treatments have been given in the past, including excision and cauterization, which can leave a scar. These practices continued until a paediatrician decided to investigate whether any treatment was necessary. He persuaded parents not to press for removal but to wait and see what happened. By this means he was able to prove that these birthmarks are harmless and that after the age of three they begin to shrink, become paler and disappear completely by the time the child is five or six years old. Any practitioner who treats a strawberry naevus is certain of success as the lesion always disappears, but it is far better to withhold treatment as this removes any danger of damaging the skin.

Orf is a skin disease caused by a virus that infects the mouths of sheep. It is most commonly found in farm workers. The human lesion is nearly always located on the hands, where it appears as a painful nodule, 2–3 cm in diameter. When I joined a GP practice in Wales, I was taught that the best treatment was to excise the skin and cauterize the nodule with a silver nitrate stick. Later, I learnt that a dermatologist had shown that this approach was not necessary as the lesion always disappears within a few weeks. The correct treatment is to reassure the patient and do nothing. This can create problems as not everyone is willing to accept such a limited approach; some people seek more active evidence of concern. The need for a 'magic' solution may explain the rationale for some of the treatments given in the Middle Ages, like the one for herpes zoster.

Herpes zoster, commonly known as shingles, is a disease most often seen in older people. It is caused by a virus. The presenting symptom is pain followed a few days later by small skin blisters similar to those of chickenpox. The blisters disappear within 2–3 weeks, though the pain is likely to persist for a long time afterwards. The lesions of shingles are always restricted to one side of the body, they never cross the mid-line. This is diagnostic. However, a remedy that I found in an ancient manuscript assumed that shingles could spread to both sides of the body, and said that if this happened the person would die.[1] The recommended treatment was to slay a lamb and with its blood to paint a cross on the sufferer's body, front and back. This was regarded as a certain means of preventing the lesions from spreading and killing the patient. It is to disprove this sort of belief and practice that scientific investigations are needed. They are also important in testing any new claims made by drug firms, healers, doctors or complementary therapists.

The Researchers

Scientific investigation of healing has been going on for some time and the subject has been widely reviewed,[2] most notably by Benor.[3] Most of the early publications were by people who were interested in psychical research and 'spiritual' healing. The first studies were mainly on simple organisms and were conducted in a laboratory setting, but eventually new patterns emerged. Researchers turned their attention to the interaction between 'healers' and their clients, then nurses explored the possibility that touch might in some way bring relief to the sick. More recently, GPs have been assessing the role of 'healers' in primary care, whilst in the United States there have been large-scale studies to see whether patients do better when they are prayed for. Various papers have also pointed out that members of certain religious sects, such as the Seventh Day Adventists and Mormons, enjoy an above-average quality of life and longevity. This chapter examines reports by scientists, healers, nurses, GPs, hospital physicians and ministers of religion: it starts with the simple laboratory tests, then moves into the clinical field, looking finally at a large-scale national study.

Experimenters often express their results in statistical terms, this is a useful guide as to how relevant they are. The terms $p < 0.05$ and $p < 0.01$ mean that the probability of the observation being due to chance is less than 5 per cent and 1 per cent, respectively. If the probability (p) is less than 0.001 the results are highly significant and most unlikely to be due to chance.

Laboratory Tests

Investigators have studied the effects of healing on a wide range of organisms, and although we are concerned primarily with the healing of people by the laying-on of hands and by prayer, a brief mention of the extent of the field is desirable. The effects that healing may have on bacteria, enzymes, plants and animals are among the subjects studied, and much of this work has been done by competent scientists in university laboratories. Bunnell chose to investigate whether healing could influence enzyme activity. Healers are reputed to produce abnormally large magnetic fields with their hands, and there is evidence that enzyme activity does respond to changes in such fields. Bunnell designed his experiment to eliminate the possibility of a placebo effect, always a confounding factor when dealing with human subjects. His purpose was to determine whether 'healing with intent' could be shown to exert an effect on the activity of the gastric enzyme pepsin. He studied the rate of breakdown of egg albumen in vitro by a 1 per cent pepsin solution using a Jenway 6051 Colorimeter at a wavelength of 470 nm. Across twenty separate trials the reaction rate of the enzyme sample 'healed with intent' by a trained healer was significantly greater than the untreated samples held by a person with no known healing abilities $(p = 0.03)$.[4]

Carol Nash set out to determine whether anybody, not just healers, could influence the growth of the bacterium *Escherichia coli*. Sixty people with no known healing ability were tested. Each person was given three test tubes containing bacterial cultures, and were asked to try to accelerate the growth of bacteria in one tube, to inhibit it in another and to keep the third tube as a control. At the end of the experiment, growth was greater in the 'growth-promoted' tube than in either the control or growth-inhibited tubes (p < 0.05). The results supported the belief, generally held by healers, that most people possess an innate healing ability.[5]

Experiments on Plants

There is no evidence to show that healing can affect the growth of plants, but positive results have been obtained from experiments on seeds and sprouting shoots. Scofield and Hodges studied the effects of healing on stressed cress seeds at the Department of Biochemistry at Wye College, University of London.[6] The seeds were soaked overnight in a saline solution to provide the 'diseased' samples necessary, these were then subjected to a period of healing by Geoff Boltwood, a gifted practitioner. The study was rigorously supervised and the tests were repeated six times, blind controls were instituted and the rates of subsequent germination carefully measured and compared.

In order to overcome any potential suggestions of trickery on the part of the healer, he was kept under constant observation, and immediately prior to each seed-handling operation was required to rinse his hands well with distilled water. Independent researchers undertook the preparation of the seed dishes, the randomization and coding of the dishes, and the assessment of growth. The healing appeared to be very successful and statistically the results were highly significant (p < 0.001). However, when the entire procedure was repeated and videotaped to create a permanent record, no significant results were obtained. This indicates the care that was taken in the attempt to validate the experiment.

Experiments on Mammals

Most of the studies on healing in animals have involved small mammals, particularly mice. Professor Bernard Grad pioneered this work at McGill University in the early 1960s.[7] In a controlled, blind study, he anaesthetized 300 mice and excised skin flaps of equal size from their backs. The wounds were examined daily for approximately two weeks, and during this time half the mice received healing from a well-known healer, Oscar Estebany. As the study was conducted blind, the researchers who measured the wounds did not know which mice had received healing. The results showed that the wounds of the healed mice closed more quickly than those of the control group, indicating that the healing had been beneficial (p < 0.01). [8] In a separate study, Grad made mice goitrous by withholding iodine from their diet and feeding them thiouracil. Half the mice then received healing. The thyroid glands grew in size in both the treated and the control animals as was expected, but when the mice were sacrificed and their thyroids weighed, those of the healer-treated group had grown significantly more slowly than those of the controls (p < 0.001).[9]

Therapeutic Touch

In the United States, nurses now routinely practise therapeutic touch (TT). In essence this is touch given with the intention to heal, though other definitions, such as a healing meditation, have been used to describe it. The term therapeutic touch was coined by Dolores Krieger, Professor of Nursing at New York University, who learnt the technique from a friend, Dora Kunz, an experienced healer and former president of the US Theosophical Society. Krieger studied its effectiveness and then taught it to students taking their Master's degree in nursing.

There appear to be many similarities between TT and 'the laying-on of hands', which has been practised in the Christian ministry and by the leaders of other religions for many centuries, but there are points of difference. TT developed as a research project and those practising it do not have to have any specific religious beliefs, nor do patients necessarily expect TT to improve their condition.[10] Also like *Reiki* healers, TT practitioners can use the method to treat themselves.

In 1971, Dolores Krieger decided to examine the role that TT might have in the treatment of anaemia. She knew that haemoglobin has a similar chemical structure to chlorophyll and that Grad[11] had demonstrated increased chlorophyll levels in plants given healer-treated water; she therefore thought it worth seeing whether healing might have an effect on human haemoglobin levels. She conducted three separate experiments with the well-known practitioner Oscar Estebany providing healing for the patients, and noted significant increases in their haemoglobin levels (p < 0.01). [12] This was the first scientific study of the effect of TT, and therefore of historical importance, but its findings would now be considered of doubtful scientific value.

Heidt was another early researcher of TT. She decided to see whether it could help ease the anxiety of patients attending a cardiovascular unit in New York City.[13] Using a Self-Evaluation Questionnaire, she measured the anxiety levels of patients waiting for treatment. She then divided the participants into three groups: one was given therapeutic touch, another casual touch and the third no touch at all. She reassessed the anxiety levels of the patients after the intervention. Those given TT recorded a highly significant ($p < 0.001$) reduction in anxiety after receiving it and they were also significantly less anxious than the patients who received just casual touch or no touch ($p < 0.01$).

Fergusson also reported an impressive reduction in anxiety among patients treated with TT. She designed a study to compare the effectiveness of experienced and inexperienced practitioners of TT. She asked one hundred nurses (fifty experienced in TT and fifty less so/learners) to assess the anxiety level of a patient of their choice by means of a Self-Evaluation Questionnaire. The nurses then gave TT to the patients and afterwards reassessed their anxiety levels. All the patients showed significantly reduced levels of anxiety, with the experienced nurses getting better results ($p < 0.0001$) than inexperienced ones ($p < 0.001$). [14]

Non-Contact Therapeutic Touch

The term 'therapeutic touch' implies that the practitioner makes physical contact with the patient's body. This differs from the way treatment is given by members of the National Federation of Spiritualist Healers as they do not usually touch their clients when giving healing. They simply place their hands within the patient's auric field, and therefore at a short distance from them. If this is an effective therapy, patients should be able to receive the full benefits of TT without the nurse actually touching them. This thinking led to an examination of Non-Contact Therapeutic Touch (NCTT); its efficacy was demonstrated by Janet Quinn, an American nurse, in the experiment she devised for her Doctoral dissertation.

Quinn randomly assigned sixty patients in a cardiovascular unit to a group who were given non-contact therapeutic touch (NCTT) and a control group who received no therapy. Four nurses administered the NCTT for a period of five minutes. During this time, the nurse centred herself mentally and made the decision to help the patient therapeutically. After becoming attuned to the patient's needs, she placed her hands 4–6 inches from their body, near the solar plexus and directed healing energy at that point. The control group received the same treatment but with one difference: the nurse did mental arithmetic whilst going through the outward motions of NCTT. [15] All the patients completed the A-State Self-Evaluation Questionnaire before and after the intervention. The results showed that the anxiety levels in the treated (experimental) group were considerably lower than in the control group after the procedure.

Fedoruk, another nurse, examined the value of NCTT in the care of premature babies. These babies are easily disturbed by routine handling and the level of distress can be measured using the Assessment of Premature Infant Behaviour scale. She studied the handling of seventeen babies and was able to show that when the nurse used NCTT before touching the infant, its stress levels were lower ($p < 0.05$) than the controls.[16] The controls were babies handled by nurses using no NCTT or mock NCTT. In mock NCTT a nurse untrained in the procedure mimicked the motions of NCTT before touching the babies, while simultaneously calculating simple arithmetic backwards out loud.

NCTT in the Healing of Wounds

It is not only nurses who practise NCTT. Daniel Wirth, a lawyer, designed an ingenious way of assessing the effectiveness of NCTT in skin healing in a study for his MA degree at JFK University, California. The study was blind, controlled and videotaped. He enrolled forty-four male volunteers in the experiment in which a medical doctor made an 8 mm full-thickness incision in their anaesthetized arms. They then attended a specially constructed laboratory daily for sixteen consecutive days. At each visit they placed their damaged arm through an aperture into an adjoining room where they thought a specially designed video camera would photograph the wound for exactly five minutes in order to study the energy flowing around the human body. In fact there was no camera in the room, instead there was the healer Lawrie Eden who gave non-contact healing (NCTT) to half the subjects. By the end of the experiment the wound in thirteen of the twenty-three people in the 'treatment group' was completely healed compared with none in the control group. The faster rate of skin closure in the 'treatment group' was statistically significant ($p < 0.001$) on both day 8 and day 16, the last day of the trial.[17]

Trials in General Practice

Family doctors are increasingly referring patients to counsellors and healers. This change in practice is well documented, but few assessments have been made of the outcome of such referrals. Brown conducted a pioneering study at his practice in West Sussex.[18] He and his partners invited patients with chronic complaints to attend a healing clinic at the practice surgery. Forty-seven people aged 16–74 were contacted and each received a leaflet explaining the rationale behind healing, and also an outline of the study. Thirty-five patients chose to attend and they received healing once a week for eight weeks, from one of two healers. Each session lasted

20 minutes. During this period a minimum time of 15 minutes was appor-
tioned to healing by laying-on of hands, with the remainder of the session
spent talking to the patient about their condition. Patients were able to
select the healer they preferred to see and, during the session, they sat
quietly in a chair whilst the healer placed his/her hands so as to 'channel
healing energies' into them. There was a relaxed atmosphere with peaceful music in the background. Most patients asked for the healing sessions
to be continued after the study was completed and this was arranged at a
time to suit the healer and the patient.

Each patient completed three SF-36 questionnaires, which provided a
good measure of their health status during the study. They completed one
before the first healing session, the next at the end of the last session and
the third six months later. Statistical calculations were performed by the
Mid-Downs District Health Authority Research Unit. Most of the referrals
were for anxiety or depression, the remainder mainly for non-specific pains.
There was no improvement in physical function, but healing did appear to
benefit patients in all the other parameters examined, resulting in improved
social function and vitality and reduced mental pain ($p < 0.001$).

Dixon published the first 'controlled' study of healing in primary care.[19]
This was a multidisciplinary trial involving a healer, a nurse, a statistician,
GPs and laboratory technicians, and it was funded by the Devon Family
Health Services Authority. The intention was to determine whether healing could help patients with intractable complaints. Dixon's partners
referred patients fitting the trial criteria to the practice research nurse.
Most referrals were for conditions associated with chronic pain. The nurse
contacted each patient by telephone, and having confirmed their willing-
ness to join the trial, allocated them to a control or treatment group. The
latter received ten weekly 40-minute healing sessions, while the controls
continued to receive only conventional care from their doctors. Fifty-seven
patients (thirty study patients, twenty-seven control) were admitted to the
trial. The healing session included time for discussion between the healer
and patient, but it mainly consisted of the healer placing her hands close
to the patient and slowly moving them over the entire body while visualiz-
ing the passage of white light through her into the patient. There was a
background of relaxing music during the session.

The research nurse assessed all the patients at the start of the trial and
again three months later. At their first meeting with the nurse, patients
recorded the intensity of their symptoms on a linear scale ranging from 0
(no symptoms) to 10 (unbearable): they also completed the Hospital
Anxiety and Depression scale and the Nottingham Health Profile, which
provides a measure of general functional ability (mental and physical). The
possibility that healing might have a beneficial effect on the immune system was also examined by determining the percentages of the natural killer

(NK) cells CD16 and CD56 in the blood at the start and completion of the survey. It was thought the interaction of the healer with the patients might alter the proportions of the NK cells though no change was noted.

Patients who received healing did better than the control group in most areas of assessment. After three months of healing, they reported an improvement in symptoms ($p < 0.05$), were less anxious ($p < 0.01$), not so depressed ($p < 0.05$) and scored better on the Nottingham Health Profile ($p < 0.01$). The results do not show whether the improvements were due specifically to the healing received or to the ambience of the session, the music and relaxation. But the conclusion reached by the researchers is that the intervention of a healer may be an effective adjunct in the treatment of patients suffering from chronic conditions.

Healing and Heart Disease

Heart disease is a major killer in Western societies today so it is not surprising that attempts have been made to assess the effectiveness of healing in the management of patients with hypertension. One such study involved ninety-six hypertensive patients and eight healers. The patients were divided equally into experimental and control groups, the former receiving distant healing whilst the controls did not. In this double blind trial neither the patients nor those conducting the experiment knew who was receiving healing. All the patients continued to take their normal medication throughout the study. Their weight, heart rate, systolic and diastolic blood pressure were monitored, and the statistical tests showed a significant drop in systolic blood pressure ($p < 0.01$) in the experimental group. The other parameters were unchanged.[20]

Another study was undertaken by doctors in the Netherlands.[21] They tested the effect of healing on 120 volunteers with hypertension, including eighty who were receiving anti-hypertensive drugs. The volunteers were allocated to three groups. Those in group 1 received laying-on of hands; group 2 had distant healing, and group 3 received no healing. Group 2 were given healing from behind a one-way mirror: this was to ensure that patients in groups 2 and 3 did not know whether or not they had received healing. This was provided by members of various Dutch healing organizations in sessions of twenty minutes once a week for fifteen weeks. There was a highly significant decrease in blood pressure ($p < 0.001$) in each group by the end of the study, but there was no significant difference between the three groups, and the experimenters concluded that the data provided no evidence that healing had an effect on blood pressure. But patients who received 'laying-on of hands' did benefit from the treatment. Of those in group 1, 83 per cent reported an increased sense of well-being compared with 43 per cent who received distant healing (group 2) and 41 per cent who received no healing. This difference between the groups was highly significant (p < 0.005), though there was no correlation between a feeling of improved well-being and a reduction in blood pressure.

Healing and Asthma

It is important to record negative findings. Johannes Attevelt found that healing offered little benefit to patients with asthma. He published his results in a Doctoral dissertation to the University of Utrecht in 1988.[22] In a carefully designed study, he tested ninety patients with asthma to assess the severity of airflow obstruction in the larger airways. He did this by measuring the *peak exploratory flow rate* (PEFR) with a peak flow meter and the *forced expiratory flow* in one second (FEV1) with a spirometer. These procedures are easy to perform with the cooperation of the patient and provide a good assessment of the severity of their disease. The patients were then randomly allocated to one of three groups. Group 1 received laying-on of hands; group 2 had distant healing from behind a one-way mirror, whilst group 3 received no healing. Changes in the recorded PEFR and FEV1 levels were used as a measure of any improvement or deterioration in function. Researchers measured the flow rates periodically in the laboratory, and the patients did so themselves at various other times at home. The equipment is easy to use and people with asthma are used to monitoring their respiratory function in this way.

Patients received eight healing/quasi-healing sessions, each lasting 15 minutes. They also continued to take any medication necessary to abort an asthmatic attack. The results indicated that there was no healing effect greater than placebo in patients in group 2 (distant healing) but there was a significant improvement in PEFR in the patients treated with laying-on of hands (group 1). An increase of 40 litres/minute was recorded at the hospital (p < 0.003) and 21 litres/minute at home. There was, however, no significant difference between the three groups as each reported improved function. Attevelt concluded that this was due to patients' expectations and the increased attention they received during the trial.

Intercessory Prayer

Intercessory prayer is a prominent part of every church service and it has an important place in the private prayers of individuals, but its effectiveness has rarely been studied and is still questioned by many people. Francis Galton's report, *Statistical Enquiries into the Efficacy of Prayer*,[23] was probably the first attempt to look at prayer objectively. It was also one of the first applications of statistics to social science. It reached the conclusion that prayer for the clergy appeared to confer no benefit on them. The report was published in 1872 and from a modern perspective the design of the survey was unsatisfactory, but it was a pioneering investigation of the subject as were two later studies on the efficacy of prayer for the sick. One was a double-blind trial with a mixed group of psychiatric and arthritic patients,[24] the other centred on eighteen leukaemic children.[25] Both trials were inconclusive, partly because the numbers involved were too small and also because the methodology was seriously flawed.

A more useful study was undertaken by Randolph Byrd. He examined the therapeutic effects of intercessory prayer on patients admitted to the coronary care unit of San Francisco General Hospital. This was a prospective, double-blind trial in which all patients admitted to the unit during a ten-month period were eligible for entry. Fifty-seven patients declined to take part: the remaining 393 patients agreed to participate and were randomly assigned to an intercessory prayer group (192 patients) or a control group (201 patients). Whilst in hospital, the first group were prayed for by Christians outside the hospital, the control group were not. The duration of hospitalization of the two groups was similar and there were no differences between the groups on admission in terms of the severity of myocardial infarction or other pertinent variables.

The intercessors were 'born again' Christians (Protestants and Catholics), who prayed daily and were active in their local churches. Each patient in the prayer group had a number of people praying for them each day. Significantly fewer patients in this group had a cardiac arrest ($p < 0.02$) or required intubation/ventilation ($p < 0.002$), or received antibiotics ($p < 0.005$) or diuretics ($p < 0.05$).[26] The results look impressive, but as Sloan and his colleagues[27] point out, the design of the trial is not completely satisfactory. The likelihood of finding statistically significant results increases when multiple statistical tests are carried out. Byrd investigated twenty-nine outcome variables, so one would expect at least one statistical test to be significant. Also, the six significant outcomes found were not independent: for instance, the prayer group experienced fewer cases of pneumonia and so might be expected to require less antibiotics: likewise it had fewer cases of cardiac failure and so received fewer diuretics. Unfortunately, these linked factors are reported separately which statisticians would find unacceptable. That said, the difference in numbers requiring intubation/ventilation is most interesting.

A similar study was undertaken in 1999 in the coronary care unit (CCU) at St Luke's Hospital, Kansas City. The research team divided 990 consecutive admissions randomly into two groups, with one group receiving remote intercessory prayer from a team of outside intercessors who prayed for each individual in the group daily for four weeks. The intercessors were predominantly women and represented a variety of Christian traditions. They did not know the patients, only their first names, and the latter were not aware that they were being prayed for in this way. More surprisingly, the staff in the CCU did not know that the trial was taking place. This unusual state of affairs was only possible because the hospital's ethical research committee had waived the requirement that staff should obtain informed consent from all patients involved in a research project. Without this waiver the trial could not have taken place.

The medical progress of the patients from the moment of hospital admission to their discharge was recorded by a CCU course score. This score ranged from 1 to 6, with a death scoring 6, a cardiac arrest 5, and the lower scores indicating a range of less serious outcomes. No difference in the length of hospitalization or stay in the CCU was observed between the two groups. However, patients in the prayer group did have a lower CCU course score, doing 10 per cent better than those in the usual care group ($p < 0.04$). The authors concluded that supplementary, intercessory prayer was an effective adjunct to standard hospital medical care.[28]

This is an important study and opens up new fields of enquiry, but there is a powerful argument against experiments of this type. It is that it is almost impossible to carry out meaningful research in this area as most patients are probably prayed for by their loved ones anyway. Supporters of intercessory prayer say that it is possible to alter the balance of prayer and that the 'prayer group' received a greater volume of prayer, perhaps even a greater intensity of focused prayer, than the controls. Whatever position is taken, the fact that there is a small but significant difference in outcome between the two groups requires an explanation, though the authors carefully avoided the suggestion of divine intervention. They drew attention to the work of James Lind who, in 1753, showed that lemons and limes cured the sailors aboard HMS *Salisbury* of scurvy without having any understanding of the role ascorbic acid plays in preventing the condition or any knowledge of the existence of vitamins. As they correctly state: 'there was a natural explanation for his findings that would be clarified centuries later, but his inability to articulate it did not invalidate his observations.'[29] Similarly, they suggest that what now appears to be healing by divine intervention may, at some later date, be seen as an outcome that had been pre-planned from the beginning by the Godhead.

Studies on Repetitive Prayer

Various studies have shown that patients do better when they are prayed for, but is prayer good for those who pray? This question was at the heart of a combined study undertaken by physicians based in four European centres: Florence, Oxford, Pavia and Gdansk. They set out to determine whether rhythmically recited prayers, like the rosary and yoga mantras, have an effect on the heart rate and blood pressure. In the study, twenty-three healthy adults recited aloud the mantra 'om-mani-padme-om' and the Latin version of the rosary prayer, Hail Mary (Ave Maria). Their mid-cerebral blood flow, ECG, respiration and blood pressure were continuously monitored during this time. It was found that the recitation in an 'alive' vibrant voice of either the Ave Maria or the mantra led to a marked slowing of the respiratory rate to around 6/minute; and a 'striking, powerful and synchronous change in cardiovascular rhythms' with a lowering of the diastolic blood pressure.

Breathing exercises are a feature of yoga practice and the recitation of mantras might have evolved as an aid to achieving a slow respiratory rate and a feeling of well-being. It is therefore not surprising that the rosary, when it is recited aloud and repetitively, can produce a similar effect and its recitation in this way might usefully be promoted as a means to good health.[30] This type of repetitive prayer is not restricted to the Buddhist and Christian traditions: the use of prayer beads is also common in Islam and it seems likely that the rosary prayer was introduced to Western society in the twelfth century by soldiers returning from the Crusades who had developed this form of prayer following their contact with the Arabs.

Prayer and Psychological Well-being

Most religious people would say that there is a correlation between a prayerful attitude to life and a sense of psychological well-being. Psychologists, on the other hand, might disagree with such a conclusion and their debate on 'whether religion is helpful or detrimental to mental well-being' is still unresolved, Maltby and two colleagues set out to determine whether there was a relationship between religiosity and psychological well-being. They started with the idea that people who claim to be religious can be divided into three groups. Members of the first group have an extrinsic orientation to religion, viewing it as a provider of consolation, protection and an opportunity to engage in group activities. Those in the second group have an intrinsic attitude to religion, living out their beliefs in their everyday lives. The third group, which Maltby calls the Quest group, consists of seekers who have an open-minded and exploratory attitude to religion.[31]

The psychologists asked 474 undergraduate students at Sheffield Hallam University to complete five questionnaires. These provided data on the religious orientation of the students, indicated whether they were clinically depressed or anxious, and gave a measure of their self-esteem. The main finding of the study was that students who pray regularly are less likely to suffer depression and anxiety than those who rarely pray. Their self-esteem is also higher and they are more likely to manage the problems of daily life satisfactorily. The frequency of private prayer, not the religious orientation of the student, is the main factor that determines the level of psychological well-being. The authors suggest that future research on the relationship between religion and the use of coping strategies in daily life should concentrate on the role of personal prayer. As Wilkinson says, 'prayer enables people to get things off their chests by talking through their problems, fears and concerns with God and derive real benefit'.[32]

Can Healing Kill Cancer Cells?

One hesitates to mention unsubstantiated claims of healing, but an interview given by Matthew Manning in *Healing Hands* has sufficient interest to merit comment.[33] He carried out his experiments on cancer cells in Texas, with the involvement of a well-known research worker, Dr William Braud, and an oncologist, Dr John Kmetz. The study is said to have been replicated at London University. Manning worked with cultures of HeLa cancer cells (the name of the cells is derived from that of Henrietta Lacks, a young woman who died from cervical cancer in 1951). Research on laboratory preparations obtained from her cells has continued for many years and has contributed to countless biomedical discoveries. This work has raised important ethical and legal issues, however, as neither Henrietta Lacks nor her family gave permission for her cells to be used in this way, and her family has never received any benefit from the profits made from them. Eventually, this contentious issue will have to be resolved in the courts.

Matthew Manning set out to see if he could destroy cancer cells by an act of will directed through his hands, which, during the experiment, he held two metres away from flasks containing the cultures. For each run three flasks of HeLa cells were prepared and the experiment was repeated thirty times. At no time was Manning in the room alone. One flask was used for the experiment: the other two were controls, one being kept in a separate room. He was allowed twenty minutes for each attempt with another person in the same room mimicking all his movements with one of the control flasks.

The effectiveness of Manning's intervention was determined by counting the cancer cells that became detached from the main body of the culture and floated to the surface. This was considered a proper test as the electrostatic charge of a cell is weakened when damaged, and this allows the cell to become detached from the main mass of tissue and float freely upwards. In twenty-seven of the thirty trials, there was a dramatic increase in the number of free-floating cells in the experimental flask, whilst there had been no change in either of the two control flasks. The importance of this experiment does not depend on the result, as many questions need to be answered about the design of the study, but on the fact that it shows that researchers can examine the efficacy of healing techniques in a laboratory using cultures of cancer cells. I was interested to hear recently from a healer who has been in contact with Matthew Manning for some years that they both find that their left hand is more effective in healing than their right.[34] I cannot speculate on why this should be so.

National Study in the United States

Between April 1996 and June 1999, the Revd Bobbie McKay and Lewis Musil undertook a national survey of spiritual healing in the United States.[35] They based their study on a random, matched sample of twelve Catholic churches and 101 churches within the United Church of Christ (UCC), a Protestant denomination of great diversity. The UCC has over 6,000 member churches and embraces both the conservative and evangelical wings of the Protestant tradition, so the sample is particularly rich in its range of responses.

The study revealed a considerable interest in healing in both the Catholic and Protestant traditions. Of the 2,200 people contacted, 700 reported having had a healing experience, though they avoided mentioning such things within the church for fear of being considered 'crazy' or 'too religious'. Some said that they had been healed of a specific disease; others reported being healed even though they had no apparent illness at the time. The latter was the healing most frequently mentioned.

In describing their experiences people often spoke of 'being changed', and by this they meant feeling simultaneously both 'better' and 'different'. The core experience was a sense of 'deep, abiding peace' and 'of knowing rather than understanding'. The moment could be recalled in great detail and frequently became a benchmark for their lives. They had difficulty in finding the right opportunity to talk of these events, so their stories were shared with only a few people and the people in whom they confided tended to be profoundly moved by what they heard. Sometimes the healing occurred in everyday situations without the involvement of any other person, and the element of surprise this engendered was apparent in many of the narratives.

After the healing many people found that their spiritual life was changed. They had a greater sense of being 'a child of God' and of being loved. They tended to be more open, gentle, patient, relaxed and non-judgemental. The 'present moment' became more important to them and increasingly they sought to serve others. These changes in attitude are very similar to those described by survivors of near-death experiences (NDEs) and one wonders to what extent the healings were linked to NDEs.

McKay and Musil found that their respondents came from all sections of the community and that they were not restricted by any credal, ethnic, geographical, gender or socio-economic boundary. They regard this as evidence that the healing experience is a natural form of ecumenicity which has the potential to become 'trans-ecumenical' in that they think the experience may be common to people of all faiths, non-Christian as well as Christian.

Retroactive Prayer

If doctors believe that prayer can benefit their patients, it is understandable that they should search for ways to optimize this effect. Many doctors regard the idea as ridiculous and Leonard Leibovici is possibly one of these, so it seems not unlikely that he may have wanted to demonstrate the absurdity of some claims that have been made when he published his paper on retroactive prayer.

Leibovici's report appeared in the Christmas edition of the *British Medical Journal*, which is traditionally a lighthearted version of this serious publication. In the year 2000 he examined the records of patients who had been admitted to an Israeli hospital between 1990 and 1996, and selected a group who had been treated for infections associated with a positive blood culture. He divided the 3,393 adults who fitted his criteria into two groups, a control and an intervention group, the selection being made by the toss of a coin. Then he gave the first name of those in the intervention group to a person who said a short prayer for the well-being and recovery of the group as a whole. An examination of the hospital records revealed that there was no significant difference in mortality between the two groups, but the prayer group had a shorter stay in hospital (p = 0.01) and a shorter duration of fever (p = 0.04).[36]

I suspect that Dr Leibovici undertook this experiment with his tongue in his cheek, almost as a joke, and that he tried the same tests with patients suffering from other illnesses such as coronary thrombosis, obtaining negative results, until he came upon this particular group of patients who happened to provide the result he was seeking. If this assumption is correct, then it was probably with a wry sense of amusement that Dr Leibovici pointed out that this type of intervention is cost-effective, has no adverse effects and should be considered for clinical practice. His further suggestion that more studies may determine the best way of delivering the prayer and uncover the reason for its success was also probably written in the same ironic spirit. I think we should not take this report too seriously, but the best way of refuting or confirming the results of any study is to repeat the experiment; this is the essence of the scientific method.

Should Scientific Evidence be Questioned?

The answer to this question is an emphatic yes. It is very important that the claims of scientists are carefully scrutinized: in fact, such questioning is the true basis of the discipline. The scientific approach has led to great increases in the sum of human knowledge, but men and women are not infallible and sometimes they make mistakes. This is apparent in many spheres of activity. Not every space probe escapes the earth's atmosphere, nor do we expect it to do so, despite the efforts made to perfect its construction. Similarly, errors are likely to occur in hospital laboratories where pathologists examine millions of specimens each year. Some women are well aware of this hazard having been informed, for instance, that their routine cervical smear tests were negative only to learn, months or years later, that cancerous lesions had been present.

The correct scientific attitude is one of constant questioning. The need for this approach became particularly apparent to me when I was the medical director of St Mary's Hospice. Occasionally, we found that patients who came to us with a diagnosis of terminal cancer were not terminally ill and did not have cancer. The diagnoses had been made in good faith by teams of doctors and nurses working in mainstream hospitals. Some of these instances have been reported in the *British Medical Journal*.[37]

Perhaps typical of these patients was an elderly widow who was admitted from a nearby hospital. She looked desperately ill and was bed-bound. The diagnosis of stomach cancer had been confirmed by gastroscopy and histology, and it was expected that all she needed was to be kept comfortable during the last few days of her life. She received the best of nursing care and was encouraged to take fluids. Slowly her condition improved; vomiting ceased to be a problem and she started to retain soft foods as well as fluids. She became stronger, put on weight and a few months later was happy and fit.

By this time it became important to suppress any suggestion that a miracle had taken place in the hospice. The first step was to ask the referring hospital to readmit the lady for reassessment. This was done. A review of the notes showed that the gastroscopist had queried the diagnosis of cancer, suggesting instead that the lesion was a large benign ulcer. However, the patient's poor physical state and the pathologist's report that the stomach scrapings were cancerous seemed to confirm the diagnosis. A repeat gastroscopy showed that the ulcer had healed completely, and when the histological evidence was reviewed by senior pathologists no evidence of cancer was found. It should be added that the pathologist who had mistakenly diagnosed cancer was herself suffering from multiple sclerosis, was working alone and had made other errors of judgement.

The patient and her family now had a new problem. Some months previously, they had come to terms with the idea of her imminent death; now they had to readjust to the likelihood that she had some years of active life ahead of her. From their perspective, her recovery had been miraculous and a certain sense of wonder remained even though there was a rational explanation for it. Is it possible that there is a rational explanation for all miracles or is it more likely, as Islam teaches, that some can be explained and others not? My patient was healed by the care and devotion shown to her in the hospice, but in what way did this influence her condition? After all, she received no specific treatment for it. We shall examine some of the possible ways this might have come about in the next chapter.

Chapter Nine
How is Healing Achieved?

Anyone who starts with the premise that paranormal sources of energy can affect the healing process must consider the possible ways in which this might come about. They should always bear in mind that one of the marvels of nature is that all living organisms are designed to protect and heal themselves. No one really heals anyone else; healers merely help a process that is innate within us and even orthodox medical practitioners merely assist this regeneration. The body is constantly renewing itself and this process of recuperation goes on all the time. The cellular constituents of the blood are replaced every few months and the bulk of the body every seven years.

If a bone is broken, provided the fracture is 'simple' and the broken ends well aligned, no outside help is needed. The body responds to the injury by mobilizing its own resources. This will involve an increased supply of blood to the injured site and an increased output of specialized cells, some to remove damaged bone particles and others to repair the fracture by laying down new bone. Scar tissue will also be formed to cover the wound. All of this happens in a coordinated way and resembles the response of a modern state when disaster strikes the country.

It would be tempting to think that this renewal could be repeated ad infinitum, but we are faced daily by the evidence that the body ages. A person of seventy years can never have the body of a twenty year old again. We must also face the fact that however knowledgeable or powerful healers may be, they can only have a limited effect for we are all destined to die. This is part of our genetic inheritance and no one can escape from it.

Spiritual healers do make a positive contribution to patient care, but whilst the interventions by medical practitioners can be scientifically justified, those of the healers usually cannot. This state of affairs is changing and it may soon become obvious that our present failure to exploit fully this well of healing is simply due to our instinctive rejection of the unexplainable. The brief accounts of the healers that I have included in this book are very compelling. In some way they were able to harness what might be called the universal life force and bring it to bear on the people who sought their help. Whether this beneficial power was absorbed by the aura or through the *chakras* I do not know, but it is probable that it had a profound influence on the body's natural defence, and recuperative, systems.

The Body's Own Defences

It is helpful to think of the human body as a walled city at risk of attack. Both will be defended in depth; both have clearly visible outer defensive walls, aggressive mobile units within these fixed lines of defence and a central chain of command to direct defenders to areas that have been breached. The first line of defence in the human body is the intact skin; this, together with the mucous membranes of the respiratory and gastrointestinal tracts, forms a physical barrier to the invasion of microorganisms. Glands in the skin and eyes also secrete anti-microbial agents which give further protection, as do the acid secretions of the glands in the stomach. If this defence system is penetrated and harmful organisms gain entrance into the blood, the body's soldiers (the white blood corpuscles) are mobilized. They surround the invading bacteria and set about destroying them. The body can also call upon more specialized natural killer (NK) cells, which attack viruses and tumour cells. All this activity is known as 'natural immunity' and it takes place in all animals, including the invertebrates, but the next line of defence, 'adaptive immunity', is found only in the more highly evolved vertebrates.

Adaptive Immunity

Adaptive immunity is based on the lymphocyte, a type of white blood cell that is produced in the bone marrow of vertebrates. Lymphocytes are of two main kinds, the B-cell and the T-cell, and these usually work in tandem. They respond to the presence in the blood of substances (called antigens) that the body regards as foreign or potentially dangerous: these may be bacteria, inhaled pollen grains, foreign red blood cells or minerals. When an antigen is detected, the two lymphocytes interact with it and each other. The B-cell then secretes an antibody that attacks the antigen. Some sensitized B-cells are retained within the bone marrow; these are called memory cells and, should the same infection recur, the body is able to respond faster and more effectively than on the first occasion. It is by their ability to manipulate this most subtle line of defence that doctors have achieved one of their major successes in extending life expectancy throughout the world.

The mass production of safe vaccines has led to large populations being protected against common infectious diseases. The programme of mass vaccination is a relatively recent development, but it has enormous potential for the well-being of the world's population. The World Health Organization was able to report in November 2000 that the scourge of smallpox had been eradicated, whereas in 1967 - an average year for small-pox deaths - it had accounted for the deaths of two million people. The WHO expects to achieve the same success soon with leprosy, and with poliomyelitis by the year 2005. Its polio vaccination programme has been so effective that in 2001 there were only 537 cases worldwide a reduction of 99.8 per cent since the programme started in 1988. China was declared free of the disease in the year 2000 and the last 'imported' case of polio into the United Kingdom was in 1982.[1]

The body is a very complex organism and we have only scratched the surface of the possible defences at its disposal. The legions of T-cells which monitor the circulatory system are highly specialized: there are helper cells, killer cells and suppressor cells. They work as a team to produce what is called the cell-mediated immune response, which results in the destruction of those foreign particles that have succeeded in evading the natural immunity of the body. If the team encounters a cancerous or a virus-infected cell, the helper T-cell acts on the surface of the cell in such a way that the killer T-cell is able to destroy it. The AIDS epidemic is flourishing at present mainly because this line of defence has been hijacked by the HIV virus and so far this has defeated all attempts to produce an effective vaccine.

Scientists continue to discover new aspects of the body's immune response. Research in this field is proceeding at an ever-increasing rate and is not restricted to the way the body copes with invading microorganisms. The immune system is also affected by the many stresses that occur in daily life so that it sometimes becomes sick itself. The individual then succumbs to one of the autoimmune disorders, which include rheumatoid arthritis, ulcerative colitis and Graves' disease. Remarkably, the body seems able to mobilize its defences to combat at least one of these diseases as, even before treatment became available, a quarter of people with thyrotoxicosis went on to have a spontaneous remission. For some, though, the relief was only temporary as about 15 per cent eventually became myxoedematous.

The Immune System

There is nothing haphazard about the body's defence and reparative systems. Just as the aggressive mobile units in a walled city were subject to a central chain of command, so the blood-borne warriors in the body's immune system are directed so as to maximize their potential. The direction is vested in the nervous and endocrine systems. The three systems are interdependent; the cells of the immune system alert the hypothalamus, the control centre in the brain, to the presence of foreign bodies in the blood. The hypothalamus responds by increasing the flow of blood to the threatened area and by triggering the release of hormones from the endocrine glands, particularly the pituitary and the adrenal glands.

The hypothalamus is part of the limbic system, the region of the brain that is closely connected with the emotions and which may be ultimately responsible for a person's sense of well-being. New insights continue to emerge on how feelings are constructed and the vital role they play in the causation of disease, an obvious example being the increased mortality in men following bereavement. Since this part of the brain is sensitive to changes in the external environment and to physical and emotional stress, it is of special interest to scientists examining the effects of psychological changes on the immune system and on the body's ability to cope with disease. Investigations so far have included studies of the responses to bereavement, unemployment, caring for relatives with Alzheimer's disease, sleep deprivation, the stress of academic examinations and travelling in space.

Conflict in relationships, stress at work and poor coping skills all lead to an increase in stress hormone levels and an altered immune functioning. Psychological stress alters the balance of T-cells within the immune system, which results in a preferential commitment to an antibody response instead of a cell-mediated immune response. Whether emotional factors play a part in the course of autoimmune disease, cancer and infectious diseases in animals and humans is a subject of intense research that has not yet been satisfactorily resolved, but we know, for instance, that almost two-thirds of patients with irritable bowel syndrome have reported an adverse life event prior to the onset of symptoms. Psychiatrists recognize that stress will respond to therapy, but few resources are available to address this component of the disease process. Experience with battle casualties shows that stress-related disorders can be resolved, but help needs to be given immediately to be effective and requires a more proactive approach than just listening and counselling. At present we cannot provide a clear explanation of why the pattern of stress-related disorders has changed over the past century. Irritable bowel syndrome has become a common complaint and so has myalgic encephalomyelitis (ME), but hysteria, a neurosis associated with emotional instability, is rarely diagnosed nowadays, though it was often seen in Victorian and Edwardian times.

To summarize this section, we may say that if a physical mechanism is required to explain the dynamics of spiritual healing, the hypothalamus and the immune system are likely to be closely involved in the process.

Esoteric Concepts

Most healers are not concerned with the working of the immune system or the role of the hypothalamus, but they are very interested in learning how to influence the energy fields that animate and surround the individual. Whilst accepting the truth of our summary of the way the body responds when under attack, they work from a different standpoint and think in terms of auras and *chakras*, of an all-pervading life force and of fields of energy that permeate the body. These ideas are not totally at odds with conventional medical thinking: scientific medicine has a good understanding of the electrical fields within the human body and has used this knowledge for diagnostic purposes for over eighty or so years. The electrocardiogram is the best known of these diagnostic aids. It is a record of the electrical activity of the heart and provides clear evidence of any damage to the structure or the functioning of that organ. Studying electrical fields in this way is a normal part of medical practice, but it is not so easy to demonstrate the existence of the energy fields used by healers. Nevertheless, many people are convinced that such fields do exist and can be recharged during a course of healing.

The Life Force

A prevailing idea behind spiritual healing, and most complementary therapies, is that an energizing force circulates within and around the body and that this can be manipulated to improve health. Often regarded as an Oriental concept, the idea is not new to the West and was taught by Hippocrates (c 460–370 BCE) and later by the Swiss physician Paracelsus (1493–1541). It gained a renewed popularity during the eighteenth and nineteenth centuries, mainly through the efforts of Anton Mesmer (1734–1815), a Viennese physician, and the German physician, Samuel Hahnemann (1755–1843). Mesmer was a great advocate of hypnosis as a method of healing. In those days hypnosis was called animal magnetism and it was generally believed that cures were effected by an occult force which flowed from the therapist into the patient. This 'animal magnetism' was regarded as a subtle, universal force of cosmological significance, which was present in all animated bodies. This belief persisted until the 1880s when it became generally accepted that there was nothing magical about hypnosis and that the trance was just a psychologically induced state in which the subject showed a heightened response to suggestion.

Hahnemann is best known for establishing the principles of homeopathy. Like Mesmer, he taught that a vital principle animates and pervades the body and that disease should be seen as a derangement of this immaterial *vital principle*. Surprisingly, Friedrich Engels (1820–95) the philosopher and collaborator of Karl Marx, held similar views. The question arises, what happens to this vital principle at death? Engels, as befits the founder of dialectical materialism, asserted that an individual's life ends at the moment of death, leaving nothing but the body's chemical constituents: dust to dust and ashes to ashes in fact. But he had to confront the problem of the vital principle – what we would call the soul – which animated the body, and accepted that it must persist. He came to the conclusion that when a person dies the vital principle merges with the Soul of All.[2] Strangely enough, this echoes the Shinto belief that, at death, a person's soul disintegrates and merges with the Universal Soul unless the appropriate rituals have been performed which enable it to retain its individuality and become a *kami*, a deified spirit.

The idea that a vital principle animates the body and that disease is essentially a derangement of this vital principle was discussed with great vigour in both medical and religious circles in the nineteenth century. This was a period when homeopathy and mesmerism flourished and for some clergymen the underlying principle acquired the status of 'a religious cause', which they could use to counteract the scientific Darwinism of the more prominent physicians. The strength of their commitment to the cause is perhaps illustrated by the statement which American clergy issued in support of homeopathy. They wrote:

> Religion itself had undergone a spiritual revolution since the date of its discovery . . . and that if homeopathy became the only medical method then for the first time will the Gospel of the Kingdom of Grace be preached and received as God ordered it to be received.[3]

One wonders if religious beliefs and medical practices will be so hotly disputed in the twenty-first century, but the practice of homeopathic medicine has endured the test of time and with osteopathy, chiropractic, acupuncture and herbal medicine is regarded as one of the 'Big Five' of complementary medicine. It is also worth noting that the nineteenth-century founders of osteopathy and chiropractic both believed in the existence of a 'vital force' that could cause disease if its normal flow was impaired.

Ch'i, Prana and Acupuncture

Belief in an all-pervading vital force is evident in many Eastern philosophies and forms the basis of some well-known traditional medical practices, including acupuncture. So it is not surprising that traditional Chinese acupuncturists have a different perception of the human body from that of Western practitioners. Whilst we tend to think of the body as a solid structure with circulating blood and hormones, they concentrate on the body's subtle energies and the pathways that facilitate the flow of *ch'i* (or *Qi*) through the living organism. Hindus call this energy *prana*. Both terms are very ancient and are often translated simply as 'breath', but whilst the Chinese *ch'i* and the Sanskrit *prana* do carry that meaning, they also refer more specifically to the primordial force that animates the universe. This force is subject to constant change and is able to appear in many guises. Just as electricity can flash through the sky as lightning, or activate various household gadgets or be the means by which impulses are transmitted along the nerves, so *ch'i* and *prana* can move through space, illuminate the stars and enliven the minds and hearts of people here on earth.

According to Eastern teaching, this energy flows through the body along set pathways or channels. Traditional acupuncturists call these channels meridians and recognize twelve pairs on each side of the body. If, as sometimes happens, the flow of *ch'i* is obstructed and it stagnates, ill-health may follow and practitioners then seek to re-establish the flow, and thereby improve the health of the patient, by inserting needles at appropriate sites on the meridians.

Traditionally, the treatment involves the use of nine types of needle. Some are like scalpel blades, but in Western practice only fine gauge needles are used, as the insertion of the larger ones can cause unacceptable pain.[4] The depth of insertion depends on the site, being greater in the more muscular areas and shallowest where the skin is close to bone or cartilage. Normally, the needles are inserted at an angle and left in place for 20–30 minutes, though for some ailments they may be left *in situ* for just 10–60 seconds. Once inserted, a needle may be twisted or twirled by hand, or connected to a source of low-voltage alternating current.

Acupuncture is a popular therapy in the West and it is becoming increasingly part of the armoury of doctors and physiotherapists, but the theoretical basis on which they offer this treatment differs from that of the traditional practitioner. They do not ascribe the beneficial effects to the manipulation of *ch'i* but to the release of endorphins, the morphine-like painkillers that the body produces when stressed. Whatever the underlying mechanism, acupuncture can be an effective analgesic and patients often notice an increased sense of well-being after treatment.

In Indian tradition, the *prana* flows through three main channels, which run along the length of the body from the nose to the perineum. These are depicted as a central column and two spiral channels that embrace it; I find this concept of particular interest as it is similar to the structure of the *caduceus*, the traditional symbol of the healing profession. This triple channel provides the central axis connecting the *chakras*, specialized psychic centres that are situated within the aura.

Aura

Most of those providing alternative therapies will probably have a different view of the human condition than that of Western-trained doctors and nurses. Practitioners offering hands-on healing are likely to be aware that they are not dealing just with the physical body, or even with the client's mental, emotional and spiritual problems; they see themselves as being involved in some unexplained way with the patient's subtle energies, fields of force that surround and penetrate right into the physical body. The innermost field is called the etheric body. This flows around the physical body and extends for about 3–4 inches beyond the skin. It is the innermost of five energy fields, which together form the aura. These other fields have their own separate functions, which need not concern us here, except to say that they are intimately linked together both functionally and structurally.

Relatively few people claim to be able to see the human aura. Those who do say that it is egg-shaped and that every individual is enveloped in one. It is part of the living condition of all organisms including plants and animals. Auras are very colourful and pulsate with energy in those who are healthy. No two auras are identical, their colour and size depend on the individual and the auras around children are noticeably different from those of adults. The colour and texture of a person's aura are not fixed; they change with any major fluctuations in thought, mood or health. This may be likened to the way a person's fingerprint is quite specific for that individual but the outline may be blurred if the hand is covered with mud.

The human aura is an accepted feature of Christian art. This is most evident in the depiction of holy men and women when their heads are framed by haloes. This practice is not restricted to paintings, such as those beautiful illustrations in the early Gospel manuscripts, it is also a feature of the mosaics that adorned ancient Christian foundations, notably the basilica at Ravenna, built in c 520.

Some people train themselves to see auras, and attempts have also been made to capture the image objectively. In 1911, Dr William Kilner, of St Thomas's Hospital used coloured screens and filters for this purpose, and Semyon and Valentina Kirlian developed a method of photographing auras which initially aroused much interest. There was a great deal of speculation about the potential of Kirlian photography for the early diagnosis of disease, especially cancer, when Sheila Ostrander and Lynn Schroeder wrote of it in their book *Psychic Discoveries behind the Iron Curtain*[5] in 1970, but it is rarely mentioned nowadays. It seems likely that the high expectations that were raised were never realized and this approach has now slipped into obscurity.

I am not clairvoyant and cannot see auras, but I understand that the ability to do so can be nurtured. Various methods for acquiring this facility are
described in the many books written on the subject. One is to gaze intent-
ly at one's reflection in a mirror with the eyes partly closed. I think that a
former patient, who was a retired nurse, had probably followed this advice.
She would discuss such matters with me and would sit with her eyes par-
tially closed when visiting my surgery, with the obvious intention of
examining my aura. Sometimes she would tell me what she saw but as this
was thirty years ago my aura would probably look quite different today. She
and her husband are both dead now, but I remember her well, partly
because they gave me a Bible when I left the area and this reinforces my
memory of them.

The Subatomic World

The precise nature of the vital healing energy that can flow through the
aura and *chakras* has not been established. This may be one of its strengths
as it provides a scenario that seems to be firmly rooted in human experience yet remains sufficiently flexible to allow for cultural variations. It fits
in remarkably well with the teachings of modern physics, which took an
enormous leap forward in 1900, when Max Planck set out his theory of
quantum mechanics and the subatomic world became the prime field for
scientific exploration. There were further developments in the mid-1980s
when the string theory was advanced, which might reconcile the previously incompatible elements of physics, general relativity and quantum
mechanics, which deal with the universe in its largest and most minute
aspects. The implications of the theory have a bearing on our perception
of space. Most of us take for granted that there are just three spatial dimensions – height, breadth and depth – but this is not so according to string
theory; it claims that our universe has many more dimensions than meets
the eye.[6] This idea is inherent in the teaching of analytical psychology. Its
founder, Carl Jung, constantly emphasized that the unconscious psyche is
not restricted by space and time, and that it possesses better sources of
information than the conscious mind which has only sense perception to
inform it.

The subatomic world is often described as a miniature galaxy with elec-
trically charged particles (electrons) revolving, like planets, around
minuscule suns (the atomic nuclei) in relatively large areas of space. All
these minute particles, and the galaxies themselves, are held together by just
four different forces. The best known of these is gravity, which surprisingly
is also the weakest natural force known to man. Gravity holds the solar

systems together and prevents people from spinning off the surface of the world into space, but its effect at the subatomic level is so negligible that it is completely ignored. The four forces that scientists have identified are, in increasing order of strength, gravity, the weak force, the electromagnetic force and the strong force. Little is known about the weak force except that it mediates radioactive decay, but we know that the electromagnetic force keeps negatively charged electrons in orbit around their nuclei and enables atoms to join together to form molecules. The strong force holds the nucleus of the atom together. It is called the strong force because it is the strongest force known in nature; it also has the shortest range known in nature, its activity being confined to the nucleus of the atom. Before 1900, the atomic nucleus was seen as an unreactive entity, but it is now known to be an arena of constant change with the continuous emission and reabsorption of particles (quarks, bosons and fermions), which can rapidly change into different types of particle at a speed approaching that of light, but only within the restricted area of the strong force.

Electrons, protons and neutrons are the best known elementary particles but neutrinos are the most widespread particles in the universe. These are subject only to the weak force and are so small and move so fast that they are constantly passing straight through the earth, and the human body, at the speed of light. The fact that such entities do exist, and that there are almost imperceptible fields of force which continue to be discovered, strengthens the beliefs of many people in the reality of the vital force which they say is essential for life and health. They believe that a block in the individual's supply of energy can cause sickness, but this fault can be corrected by an inflow of healing energies from another person.

One of the best-known examples of the transfer of this force is told in the story of Jesus healing the woman with a haemorrhage. When she touched him he immediately asked, 'Who touched me?' and later said, 'Someone touched me; I know that power has gone out from me.'[7] Some healers speak of this vital energy as a fifth force, which they believe will eventually be detected by scientific instruments,[8] and it is perhaps pertinent to point out that the existence of the weak force was only demonstrated quite recently and we still do not know much about it.

Learning about the Aura

Children are not taught about the aura at school and the subject was not included in the curriculum at my medical school. People acquire this information from other sources and my introduction was effected by a Jesuit priest, Fr Andrew Glazewski. Our contact was brief and took place at a residential course which I had joined in the expectation that the main theme would be on death and dying, two aspects of existence that then interested me. But Andrew's introductory session was on the subtle energies that radiate from all living organisms and how it was possible to detect these forces through the palms of the hands. The technique is broadly similar to the one used by dowsers and my first practical lesson came later, when a farm worker showed me how he detected underground water by dowsing with hazel sticks. However, Andrew was mainly concerned in showing us how to become attuned to plants and trees.

I learned something else. During his opening discourse, it was obvious that he was not well. He would lean for support on the back of a chair that was placed in front of him for that purpose, and his friend, an Anglican priest, sat alongside him with his arms outstretched, the palms directed towards the speaker. This looked weird but its significance became clearer later.

When the evening session was over, I was among the last to leave the room. Andrew was talking to a few friends who seemed concerned about his health, so I asked how he was and was told that he had angina and that during the lecture he had experienced pain in the back of the neck. He said the pain was easing, so I went to bed. About twenty minutes later there was a knock on the door and I was told that Andrew was not well and was asked if I would come and see him. I found him lying on his bed, dead. We did not try to resuscitate him, but said some prayers and informed the coroner's officer and the Abbot of nearby Prinknash Abbey. I realize now that the Anglican priest had been trying to support Andrew with healing energies. His efforts did not save Andrew's life, but they may have helped him to complete his lecture. Since then I have seen many people die, and some deaths have been most beautiful, but none has shown me so clearly how to walk boldly into the next world.

When I returned home, I naturally discussed the weekend's events with my wife, Valerie. I was particularly keen to share with her my new understanding of the energies surrounding plants, but she received the information with almost quiet indifference, merely informing me that she had always been aware of such forces and that they affected her most strongly when she stood under trees. Before that moment, I had not the faintest idea that she had ever had such experiences, though we had been married for over twenty years. Later, with their consent, I used to explore the energy fields surrounding my patients using a stethoscope as a dowsing aid. The most common observation was that the field of force over a pregnant abdomen was always particularly great, diminishing abruptly after the baby was delivered.

Chakras

The aura forms just part of the subtle energy body. Within it lie the *chakras*. These are highly specialized areas that cannot be detected by the normal physical senses. Whilst the aura has always been a universal symbol, our understanding of the *chakras* is a more recent awakening and is dependent on Eastern teachings, particularly the deeper insights into the human psyche provided by eastern meditative practices. Jung believed our failure to grasp the idea sooner was due to a difference in temperament between Eastern and Western peoples. He regarded Westerners as natural extroverts who are keen to explore the outer world: in contrast the people of the East tend to be introspective and are more interested in understanding the nature of their inner psyche. There is, as a consequence, a much longer tradition of the teaching and practice of meditation in the East and it is in contemplation that one becomes aware of the *chakras*.

If a comparison may be drawn, the outgoing love of St Francis of Assisi (1182–1226) is more in tune with the Western psyche than the quiet contemplative life, in a hermitage cell, of Dame Julian of Norwich (1342–1416), but it is through inner quietness that inner realities are most readily perceived and as the psalmist said most pertinently, 'Be still and know that I am God.'[9] Withdrawal from the world and quiet devotion have always been an aspect of monastic life in the West, but the practice of meditation has only recently become part of the life of people in the West. I remember being at a healing conference many years ago where some of us were led in the 'prayer of silence' by a laywoman. It was a beautiful experience and at the end she was the first person to leave room, expecting the rest of us to follow in our own time. When the door shut behind her, a nonconformist minister immediately said, 'Now, let's have a proper prayer meeting' and at once broke into extempore prayer. The magic of the moment was shattered.

When I sit quietly in meditation, I sometimes become aware of a very definite rotatory force in the region of the heart and forehead. These forces sometimes rotate in unison, though each is quite separate from the other. They are not perceptions that I can deliberately induce and any attempt to observe them consciously causes the effect to stop. I do not know whether these are my *chakras*, but the possibility that they might be does occur to me. We are dealing with a concept that is rooted in Eastern religious teachings, and consequently it is likely to be denounced as anti-Christian in some church circles. This would be unfortunate for *chakras* have no religious significance at all. If they exist they are merely part of our psycho-spiritual condition and are no more relevant to our religious beliefs than our hearts or endocrine glands.

The Appearance of the *Chakras*

The word *chakra* comes from the Sanskrit term meaning 'wheel', and they are sometimes likened to transformers which take in the subtle energy that permeates the cosmos and distribute it throughout the body. *Chakras* are perceived as pulsating, rotating wheels of light located at seven major points in the body and at various minor ones. The major *chakras* are those at the top of the head, between the eyebrows, and at the level of the throat, heart, solar plexus, sacrum and coccyx. They form a unified complex along the length of the body and are connected by the channels through which the *ch'i* or *prana* flows. *Chakras* are not limited by the boundaries of the physical body; they extend into the space occupied by the aura, and each has its own rate of vibration – the root *chakra* rotating at the slowest rate and the crown *chakra* the highest.

Some authorities describe *chakras* in precise detail; others advise against this, regarding them not as fixed, physiological forms but as 'spiritualized, dynamic psychological' entities',[10] which vary according to the individual's spiritual development and their ability to control the flow of *ch'i/prana*. However a brief description of the more commonly ascribed attributes of the *chakras* is appropriate.

The *chakras* are sometimes said to resemble a lotus flower, which is rooted in the mud and looks to the heavens. Each has a specific number of petals; the root *chakra* is four-petalled, the one at the heart centre has twelve petals, whilst at the top of the head lies the thousand-petalled crown *chakra*. The *chakra* between the eyebrows possesses only two petals because, in Tibetan teaching, it is not considered a separate centre but part of the crown *chakra*.

When a person is in good health, the *chakras* are flexible and radiate good colours. Although it is possible for a *chakra* to emit any colour, a clear relationship does exist between certain colours and particular centres. The root *chakra* is predominantly red and the crown *chakra* violet, with the other colours of the spectrum associated with the *chakras* in between as shown in the figure. This relationship is incorporated into crystal healing and the *chakra*'s dominant colour will be an important factor for the practitioner to bear in mind when selecting crystals for healing. So too is the identification of the *chakras* with the earth elements, the musical scale and much else.

Over the many years since they were first divined the *chakras* have been accorded other relationships. For instance, the root *chakra* is said to have a special affinity with the earth, the sacral centre with water, the one at the solar plexus with fire and the heart *chakra* with air. The upper *chakras* tend to be identified more closely with the spiritual nature of mankind. The heart centre is considered to have a special role in maintaining a person's

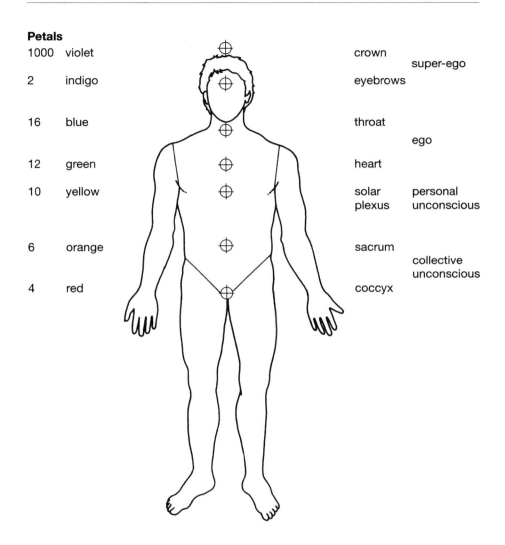

Petals

1000	violet	crown	
			super-ego
2	indigo	eyebrows	
16	blue	throat	
			ego
12	green	heart	
10	yellow	solar plexus	personal unconscious
6	orange	sacrum	
			collective unconscious
4	red	coccyx	

Figure 9.1 Relationships of the Chakras.

inner harmony and is often equated with the ego. The centre at the sacral level is said to be closely related to the personal unconscious and the lowest one with the collective unconscious.

Some healers focus on their *chakras* when meditating. For instance, a 'Meditation on the Elements' is part of the Sufi healing tradition; its aim is to strengthen and purify the *chakras*, and by this means the entire inner person, but there is a parallel intention and that is to offer a benediction on the whole of creation in both its most minute and majestic forms. This meditation focuses first on the root *chakra* where it embraces all the earth-

ly elements in the human frame and the universe. Subsequently, the meditation concentrates on the water and fire elements and at the heart *chakra*,
the air. The throat *chakra* is seen as the 'gate to the soul' and the crown
chakra as a link to the source of spiritual grace, the Godhead. Through this
last *chakra* Sufis channel divine light into their inner being so that it may
heal and purify each *chakra* in turn.

Hand Healing

The palms of the hands have always been regarded as important sources of
psychic energy, secondary only to the main *chakras* where this vital energy
is accumulated, transformed and distributed. When the main centres are
harmonized and integrated, the secondary centres, like the palms of the
hands, are capable of radiating the focused energy and transmitting it. This
is the basis of all ritual gestures, such as the act of blessing, and finds its
most distinctive expression in the 'laying on of hands'.[11] During healing
people are often aware that something significant is happening to them
and they frequently mention an increased sensation of warmth, or cold-
ness. Those who received healing from Cameron Peddie would often speak
of the 'sea breezes' that he seemed to waft towards them and of the sweet
smelling oil that appeared on his hands. Although I hesitate to do so, I feel
inclined to speak of it as an 'odour of sanctity', which was also a feature of
the healings of Hilda Ingram. It is possible that the oil mentioned by St
James in his famous Epistle with which the elders would anoint the sick
referred to a similar oily secretion on sanctified hands and not, as is the
present custom, to a vegetable oil that has been consecrated by a bishop
and then used by priests in healing rituals.

   When I place my hands close to Valerie with the intent to heal, she
always says they convey a lovely feeling, very peaceful and relaxing, and that
she feels a warm tingling glow, particularly over the head. I must admit,
however, that the sensation is never as dramatic as the one she experiences
when standing under a tree. The ability of parts of the body to concentrate
power may explain those accounts of people whose hands have emitted a
visible radiance. This is outside my personal experience, but my friend
John Mitchell still speaks of a Catholic priest whose hands radiated light
when he consecrated the host at mass. The ability of the human form to
radiate an inner light may help to explain the Transfiguration of Christ,
witnessed by Peter, James and John, and those other transfigurations that
are sometimes, though rarely, reported.

   The sick can be healed in diverse ways, with the knife, drugs, listening
skills, prayer, sympathy and with the hands, but most people who call them-

selves healers use some form of hand healing. Some work best if they have direct physical contact with the patient; others prefer the non-contact approach. Direct contact with the hands is essential in some therapies such as *Reiki*, but in *Reiki* the patient does not need to undress. They have only to loosen tight clothing and then relax in a chair or on a couch while the healer places his/her hands on the covered body. Some therapies do require the patient to remove garments. Top of this list is probably aromatherapy, as the application of oils to the skin is an essential part of the treatment; similarly a LaStone therapist can function only if she has direct contact with the skin of her client. Although direct contact with the patient is sometimes essential, therapists are not only concerned with the physical side of their client's complaints; their intention is to provide relief in an all-embracing way.

LaStone Therapy

There are many therapies that are derived from the concept of a vital flowing energy and the ability to access this through the aura and *chakras*. LaStone therapy is one of newest. It was introduced by Mary Hannigan in 1993 in the United States and the method is being taught in a number of other countries. Basically, the treatment involves the use of water-heated basalt lava stones and cold marble stones, combined with a traditional body massage, aromatherapy or hot oil treatment. The method enables the therapist to concentrate on specific lesions and provide a total body treatment simultaneously.[12] Each session lasts about 1¼ hours and begins with the client undressing and lying on hot stones, which have been covered with a towel. Stones are then placed on the abdomen and chest, on the forehead and under each arm. Tiny ones are placed between the toes and the therapist also uses stones when massaging the body, one stroke of massage with a stone being considered equivalent to ten conventional massage strokes. The aim is to combine physical and spiritual healing, and part of the therapist's intention is to open the client's *chakras*.[13]

I am not sure how that is achieved, but the positioning of polished stones on selected sites of the body is also a feature of crystal healing. In the latter, stones may be used alongside crystals and both will be chosen to infuse the aura with light and to activate the *chakras*.[14] More pertinently, crystal therapy practitioners believe that during treatment they can exorcise demonic energies and open a window into the deeper recesses of the psyche.

Spinal Touch

Spinal touch is another contact therapy. It is one of the twenty-five independent therapies that form the Association of Light Touch Therapists. Its founder was John Hurley who, in the 1920s, concluded that the chiropractors of his day did not treat the body as a unified whole and that the energy systems of the body were best influenced by a light touch. His published views[15] were reformulated in 1975 by Dr La Mar Rosquist in *The Encyclopaedia of Spinal Light Touch Treatment*. This retains Hurley's basic principle of the value of 'light touch' and the need to ensure that the body's centre of gravity is aligned through the lumbar-sacral joint, but gives greater emphasis to the care of the sacrum (literally the sacred bone) than was previously considered necessary.

The therapist starts by measuring the body's vertical axis with a plumbline. Ideally, it should fall straight down the spine through the centre of gravity at the lumbar-sacral joint. Any drift from this optimal alignment is marked in ink on the skin to guide the therapist when she is correcting distortions in the sacrum. Treatment consists of light but precise touch to various acupuncture points, reflex points and those places where muscles are attached to bones, beginning at the junction of the buttock with the thigh. By this means, we are told, spinal touch enables the body to redirect its energy so that it heals itself. Some clients are also said to experience subtle changes in their *chakras* associated with a regeneration of their energy fields.

Reflexology

Reflexology is another widely available contact therapy. The principle underpinning it was formulated by an American physician, Dr William Fitzgerald (1872–1942), popularized by his colleague Dr Bowers, who called the treatment Zone Therapy, and further developed by an American masseuse, Eunice Ingham, who introduced her own system of massage, the Ingham method of compression massage.

Reflexology is based on the idea that a vital energy circulates in a balanced, rhythmic way round the body and that, if the flow is interrupted, disease is experienced. This is similar to the views held by Hahnemann, Mesmer, traditional Chinese acupuncturists and many others, but reflexologists recognize only ten main energy channels, not the twelve meridians of Chinese acupuncture. The vital energy is perceived as flowing downwards from the head to the fingers and toes, permeating every cell and tissue. Should the flow be interrupted and disease occur, health is restored by unblocking the channels. The therapist does this by massaging the feet and applying pressure to specific areas on the sole of each foot.

Dr Fitzgerald taught that the feet, and in particular the soles, are a mirror image of the entire body. The right foot reflects the right side of the body and the left foot those organs on the left side. The same is true of the hands, but because the energy terminating in the feet is considered more powerful it is thought best to treat the patient there. I cannot comment on the effectiveness of reflexology, but I was always impressed by an elderly beautician who used to visit the hospice where I worked. She came as a volunteer and would just sit and rub the patient's hands. They always felt better for her visits and if healing can be imparted quietly and unobtrusively she did it *par excellence*.

I must say that I like to have my feet rubbed. A foot massage is a very comforting and relaxing experience, and in that sense is therapeutic, though whether the patient gains any other benefit is open to doubt. It is certainly soporific. My wife does not claim to be a healer, but she can regularly send me off to sleep in a few minutes just by rubbing my feet. As a consequence, my blood pressure is lowered and the workload of my heart is reduced. This must be helpful, even though the effect is transitory.

Learning to Heal

There has been a big upsurge of interest in healing over the past few decades and with it a huge demand for training in the necessary skills. As a consequence, schools of healing are being established with amazing rapidity throughout the world. Some are based in universities where it is now possible to take degree courses and doctorates in a range of complementary therapies, and parallel developments are taking place in medical schools. In 1994, courses in spiritual healing and complementary medicine were available in only three medical schools in the United States. This number had risen to sixty in 1999, with another hundred schools intending to introduce such courses into the curriculum. In most instances the courses are voluntary. In India, a proposal by the government to make the study of traditional medicine compulsory in medical schools has been opposed by the doctors mainly because the curriculum is too overcrowded.

Some European countries require medical students to have some knowledge of complementary medicine and most schools in the UK now provide courses dealing with a range of alternative therapies. Similar provisions are available for nurses and in the 1980s our English National Board course for postgraduate nurses at St Mary's Hospice included a module on complementary medicine. Many of the developments in the teaching and practice of CAM medicine have, in the UK, been greatly helped by The Foundation for Integrated Medicine, the brainchild of HRH the Prince of Wales. Since its foundation in 1993, progress has been made in education, research and communication between workers in this very wide field. Possibly of more significance has been the establishment of statutory regulatory bodies for osteopathy and chiropractic, and the pursuit of similar legislation to govern the practice of acupuncture and the herbal therapists.

English law allows anyone to treat a sick person but restricts the use of certain titles such as nurse, dentist or physiotherapist, which have been designated by law. Before the year 2000, anybody could claim to be a chiropractor or an osteopath if they so wished, but it is now a criminal offence to do so unless they are registered by the General Osteopathic Council (established by Act of Parliament in 1993) or by the General Chiropractic Council (established by statutory Act in 1994). This legislation came into force in May 2000 and is intended to ensure that all practitioners have proven high standards, both of clinical competence and professional conduct.

Many courses are being advertised for training in healing, but few possess the academic and professional standards provided by the universities and the schools of chiropractic and osteopathy. The governing councils of other groups in the healing sector are constantly seeking to raise their standards. In the forefront of this campaign is the Confederation of Healing Organizations (CHO) and the British Complementary Medicine Association (BCMA). The BCMA speaks for 20,000 registered practitioners of many different therapies, whilst the CHO acts as an umbrella organization for thirteen independent associations of spiritual healers. The CHO provides guidelines for the training schemes offered by each of its thirteen members, and practising students are bound by the CHO Code of Conduct. Its Healing Accreditation Course costs £900 and is arranged within five modules taken on a part-time basis over two years. Students are taught basic anatomy and physiology, and learn to connect with, and channel, the universal healing energy, the earth energy and the heart energy. Other techniques they learn include balancing the major and minor *chakras*, absent and contact heaing, working with their spirit guides, dealing with psychic attack and working with dreams.

An entirely different approach is that of the Ellel Ministries training schools. These internationally based Bible Colleges provide residential courses ranging from twenty days to six months with a special emphasis given to evangelism, deliverance and healing. The courses appear to be lively occasions, with plenty of discussion, student participation, drama, prayer, worship and individual support. The subjects studied include the Foundations of Christian Truth, the Biblical Basis of Healing, Care and Counselling, Leadership, Teaching Skills and Interculture Ministry.

Conclusion

Healers have different views about their role in relieving suffering. Some see themselves as custodians of a special gift to heal; most regard themselves as a channel, or pipe, though which the healing energy flows. The nature of this energy is also a subject for debate, not so much in terms of its effectiveness but of its origin and designation, even the name by which it should be called.

Harry Edwards believed that his healing work was done in conjunction with spirit guides, in particular with Louis Pasteur and Lord Lister, both eminent Victorians. Other spiritual healers have their own guides and many, whilst being sympathetic to such views, probably do not take them too seriously. *Reiki* healers do not give too much thought to the *vix medica- trix naturae* they channel and I imagine the same probably applies to acupuncturists and chiropractors. In Christian circles the situation can get a little fraught. All Christian healers will acknowledge that Christ is the source of their healing power, but the emphasis given to the use of His name as a healing mantra varies greatly. A member of the Society of Friends who has a healing ministry is likely to undertake this work in a quiet reflec- tive way along the lines described by Elizabeth Stubbs, who wrote:

> Contact healing is a form of sharing, of communion at a deep level of con- sciousness, through prayer, through love, through the offering of oneself as a channel for the healing power of the spirit of God, as is all spiritual heal- ing; but, with the addition of touch, and time, time actually spent physically with the sufferer where he or she is.

She goes on to say that contact healing lends itself particularly well to a healing group where there is

> a gathered and centred down silence, with or without words of healing prayer or ministry; all present being comfortably positioned, so that at the appropriate time all may take time to lay hands on the sufferer without strain, and wait, until the group is aware that the healing is finished for that session.[16]

The ministry provided by the Trelowarren Fellowship is probably just as effective, but its approach is different. The Fellowship's healing is firmly based on Bible teaching and they always pray in Jesus' name. This is central to their ministry because, as a member of the Fellowship pointed out to me, there are faith healers who are not Christian, but those who are Christian believe that Jesus is the Healer and the healing comes in His power, so His involvement must be acknowledged by using his name.

We can define Christian healing in many ways, but in essence it is the renewal of our relationship with Christ. Bishop Morris Maddocks put it this way: 'Christian healing is Christ meeting you at your point of need.' The Director of the Christian Healing Mission, John Ryeland, says, 'Healing is about us becoming like the vision that God has for each of us' and adds, 'I once heard someone say, Jesus loves us just the way we are, but he loves us too much to let us stay that way.'[17] The Director of Cautley House, the Revd Patrick Jones, puts it differently: 'The Christian Healing Ministry is a ministry of love which relates to the whole person, to every aspect of life – body, mind and spirit.'[18]

All these definitions imply a harmonious relationship with the eternal, well expressed in the Hebrew word shalom which Dr Peter Ashton tells us implies more than just peace as we use the word. He says:

> It describes a sense of well-being, good health, happy relationships and salvation where God's will is being done and fulfilled. Inevitably this means a change of heart and of direction for we are prone to wander from our Father. It implies the recognition of our relationship with God that he longs for, and which for the Christian can only be achieved through Christ. So again we come back to healing as the restoration of a relationship with God without which we can never be whole. It is Jesus who makes it possible.[19]

So the 'whole' person is one who is in harmony with their Maker. It is perhaps the emphasis placed on the pivotal importance of achieving this goal that is behind the modern obsession with deliverance therapy. It is difficult to give an objective assessment of such an emotive subject, but it cannot be ignored as, increasingly, those attending church healing services will be confronted by the challenge that they are possessed.

Chapter Ten
Healing by Deliverance

Deliverance is the modern term for the casting out of demons. The idea that the sick can be healed in this way is, for the most part, quite alien to modern Western thinking, but this entrenched attitude is gradually being undermined, certainly since I qualified as a doctor in 1956. Then, the churches were not concerned greatly with healing or with deliverance, which was then called by its traditional name, exorcism. Now the situation is different: as the Church's commitment to healing grows, so its interest in demons and deliverance seems to burgeon. This is apparent in various ways. For instance, bishops are authorizing increasing numbers of priests to act as exorcists, the output of academic books and reports on the subject is increasing and, inevitably, exorcism has become a source of comment to the media. Within the past thirty years, the Church of England alone has produced the Exeter Report (1972),[1] the York Report (1974)[2] a handbook by the Christian Deliverance Study Group (1986)[3] and a chapter on 'Deliverance' in *A Time to Heal* (2000),[4] the detailed report on the Ministry of Healing commissioned by the English bishops. In their support of the practice of exorcism in 1975, the General Synod of the Church of England gave the following ruling.

> there are many men and women so within the grip of the power of evil that they need the aid of the Christian Church in delivering them from it. When this ministry is carried out the following factors should be borne in mind:
>
> 1. It should be done in collaboration with the resources of medicine.
> 2. It should be done in the context of prayer and sacrament.
> 3. It should be done by experienced persons authorized by the diocesan bishop
> 4. It should be followed up by continuing pastoral care.[5]

It would be helpful if all the details of this ruling were followed precisely, but this is not always the case. I have heard worrying reports that an

165

increasing number of people are being told at Christian healing services that they are possessed by demons. This accusation is directed at those who have a problem with alcohol or drugs, who are homosexual or lesbian, who masturbate and are anxious, and to people whose families have been associated in any way with Freemasonry or Spiritualist churches. We are also told that there is evidence of demonic activity in almost half of all those who have been widowed and that 55 per cent of nurses have been involved in occult practices which lay them open to demonic influences.[6]

Non-Christian Exorcism

It is not only the Christian Churches that practise exorcism. It is also a feature of the religious traditions of many cultures. This point is recognized by John Richards in his booklet *Exorcism, Deliverance and Healing*, where he makes a distinction between 'Christian exorcism and non-Christian exorcism'. He says:

> Various occult groups, spiritualists, etc. can and do exorcize. Christian exorcism is that undertaken in the name of Christ operating by his Holy Spirit within his Church.[7]

Therapeutic non-Christian exorcism has been mentioned briefly in Chapter 2, and specific instances of its use have been cited for Indonesia, India, Puerto Rico, the Philippines, northern Sudan and other parts of Africa. This is not a comprehensive list and merely indicates the extent of the practice. Exorcism has a long tradition and 2,000 years ago Jesus and his disciples cast out many demons, though there is no mention of the subject in the earlier records of the Jewish people. It is worth noting also that exorcism has been part of the funeral rites of the Japanese emperor and his family for over a thousand years.[8]

Expelling demons is not part of normal medical practice, nor does it usually feature in complementary medicine, but it is to be found in some forms of alternative medicine. Katrina Raphael, for instance, has discussed its place in crystal therapy. She describes two distinct types of demonic force that can afflict the individual. The first results from our negative thoughts and habits, which can influence our conscious decisions. She believes that these tendencies can become so powerful that they behave as living entities within us and can cause us to act as if we are under the possession of an alien force.

The pervasive influences of the traditional 'seven deadly sins' — anger, gluttony, lust, pride, sloth, avarice and envy — would belong to this category. A crystal therapist would deal with these challenges by helping her client to develop their own strength of will and by activating the light force within the subtle body through the correct use of crystals.

The other type of demon she mentions is encountered less frequently. This is an outside entity, which gains entry into the aura of a susceptible individual and feeds on their vital energy. Her advice to the therapist in dealing with these forces is to claim complete authority over them and command them either to integrate with the person's purpose or to depart, and never to return. Raphael believes that crystal healing is a very effective way of dealing with demonic forces.[9]

In these scenarios the distinction between Christian exorcism and non-Christian exorcism is easily seen. The situation becomes a little more blurred when we consider the healing rites of what might be termed heretical Christian Churches. The Church of Jesus Christ of Latter-Day Saints would probably fall into this category. Mormons exorcise demons and do so in the name of Jesus Christ. The question arises, is this a Christian exorcism or something different? Other questions need to be considered. For instance:

• Is Christian exorcism more effective than non-Christian exorcism?
• If it is considered more effective, what is the evidence to support such a claim?

Sometimes it is easier to pose the questions than come up with the answers. I would have to reply to both the above 'I don't know', but this is a field of enquiry that an independent researcher could usefully examine.

Deliverance and Evil

When we consider 'deliverance', the casting out of demons, we are faced by one of the big questions which confronts thoughtful people: What is the nature of evil and what is its source? Of its existence there is no doubt. The seventy-three years of my own lifetime have witnessed the Second World War, the Holocaust, the Soviet Gulags, civil wars in Africa, Asia and South America, genocide in Cambodia, Rwanda and Central Europe, famines and the importation into the West of so many narcotics that 50 per cent of our young people have taken illicit substances. Most of us are also aware of the propensity for evil within ourselves. No one remains untainted, not even our foremost religious leaders, evangelists and exorcists. It is because they help us to cope with our inner frailty that the teachings and rites of our chosen religion are so important.

Among the aspects of human nature that we castigate as bad are our anxieties and fears, illicit sexual cravings and hatred of others. These feelings often arise unbidden and their sudden eruption into our conscious mind make them difficult to handle. Depth psychologists believe they originate in the 'unconscious' where the archetypes and 'shadow personalities' of the individual are found. This intriguing idea makes good sense, but few people have the opportunity or inclination to study such matters in detail. A more conventional explanation is provided by personifying evil in the form of the Devil, and his/her minions, the demons.

A belief in the power of demonic forces can be overwhelming as I discovered when I was providing a counselling service at a large parish church. On one occasion, I was told that a young man was seeking 'spiritual advice' and it was hoped that I might be prepared to see him. Of course I agreed, and after the initial introductions we went to a small chapel where we could speak in private, yet be open to the public gaze.

Brian had many problems but was fortunate in having a good job, a comfortable home and a good relationship with his wife. He was very restless and early in the conversation wanted to know if I believed in the Devil, to which I answered 'no', though I did believe in the reality of evil. This answer seemed to give him some comfort, but he remained restless and worried. Then he started to talk more easily and described how, when he was living with his in-laws, he had seen the ghost of an old woman and called his wife, but all she saw was a dissolving mist. No one else had noticed anything unusual, but the experience continued to trouble him even after they had moved into their own home.

Subsequently, his brother was brutally murdered and his father-in-law died. He always felt that the 'old man' was never given a proper burial, he was just cremated and his ashes buried in a garden. There was now a pause in his flow of talk and he wanted to know if I believed in hell, and I said 'no', though I firmly believed in an afterlife. This reply also seemed to help as it was pertinent to one of his more immediate problems. A few days before he consulted me, he had returned home and detected a burning smell in the house, a smell that he associated with his father-in-law. This had really frightened him as he believed that the dead man had come back from hell, as a demon, to harm him.

If I had been a priest I might have chosen to exorcise him and he would have gone away feeling better, but reinforced in the belief that demons do exist and can inflict harm on us mortals. As it was, he went away very elated because his fears had been dealt with. He no longer saw the dead as wielders of demonic power and he took with him a strengthened assurance that his brother was in heaven. He left so buoyantly I had no opportunity to share with him the short prayer which, in that particular setting, would have been appropriate.

That was not the end of the saga, I was asked to see him again a few weeks later and found him distressed with other problems that he needed to share.

He could not sleep and his doctor had put him off work but he was not taking the tablets he had been prescribed. We had another long session during which I listened while he talked about his worries and fears, and this time we finished with a prayer which simply commended him to the love and protection of Jesus. He left saying he felt much better and able to cope.

Major and Minor Exorcism

The Christian Church has a long tradition of distinguishing between two types of exorcism. These it calls the major (or greater) and the minor (or lesser) exorcisms. The former is rarely performed and, in episcopal churches, the person conducting this exorcism normally needs the bishop's permission to do so. The central act of a major exorcism is a direct command, given in the name and power of Christ, to the demon or demonic forces to depart from that individual or place forever, to go to their own place, and not to harm any human being (alive or dead) as they depart. Some liturgical guidelines for this form of service have been published by Richards.[10]

The lesser exorcism is invoked more frequently. It forms part of the baptismal service and is also used in the blessing of water, oil and sacred vessels. It does not presume a state of possession, but is essentially a rejection of evil together with prayers asking for its power to be negated. This is part of the normal pastoral work of the ordained Christian minister, though any Christian may act as an exorcist if the situation warrants it. The Lord's Prayer with its petition 'deliver us from evil' is a minor exorcism that is in common usage. To quote the Christian Deliverance Study Group, 'A minor exorcism is a prayer to God, whilst a major exorcism is a command to an unclean spirit.'[11]

The Practice of Deliverance

Those who believe in the possibility of demonic possession do not agree on how often it might occur. Some say it happens only rarely, others see evidence of possession in people suffering from medical disorders such as epilepsy, and in the bereaved when they feel their loved ones to be close to them. These people are not possessed but, depending on the Christian groups they encounter, they may find themselves the focus of a ritual act of deliverance.

Christianity has many different sects and denominations, and the frequency with which exorcism is practised varies between these different groups. It is unlikely, for instance, to be a feature of Quaker meetings, or even practised by any member of the Society of Friends. In contrast, it would not be considered unusual in some Pentecostal churches nor would the youth of the person believed to be possessed be regarded as a reason for withholding the ritual. This differs from the position adopted by the Church of England, which normally excludes 'young children and animals' from this ministry.[12] This ruling raises the question: 'At what age are young children likely to suffer demonic possession?' And: 'If it is an effective ministry, why should it be withheld on the basis of age?'

Two different approaches to deliverance were portrayed recently on English television. One was the exorcism of a child in a charismatic fundamentalist church. Here, although the cameras were privy to the preceding deliberations, they were not allowed to witness the act itself. What was apparent, however, was that the proceedings were noisy, lively and lengthy. It is difficult to imagine what effect this would have on the child who was probably not more than six or seven years old.

The other film featured the Revd Tom Willis, one of twelve exorcists licensed in the Diocese of York. Tom is a retired parish priest who is asked to investigate about twenty-five cases of occult disturbance each year. Most of these seem to involve 'the restless dead'; he deals with very few cases of possession, maybe one every 2–3 years, and even then he is not sure that these people are actually possessed. He comes across as a gentle, quietly spoken, Guinness-drinking priest, who relates well to distressed people. Although he shares the work with other priests, and they meet on a regular basis with the bishop, he tends to work alone and, in reaching a diagnosis, seems largely dependent on the reports provided by eye witnesses.

The film showed Tom Willis exorcising two houses in Hull. The people living in the houses were obviously very distressed and there was no doubting their belief in the presence of evil spirits, or their conviction that exorcism might help. His technique was quite simple. He walked through each house, telling the lost spirits to depart and blessing everyone, including the pets, using holy water to place the sign of the cross on the walls of each room.[13] Both families benefited from his ministrations. One felt more peaceful, the other was rehoused by the council.

The Devil

Of the existence of evil there is no doubt, but are we justified in ascribing it to a personalized demonic force, to an individual usually known as Satan or the Devil, and if so how did humanity come to this conclusion? The conflict between good and evil is a central drama in the folk stories, myths and religions of all cultures but in the Judaeo-Christian-Islamic tradition it first appears in the book of Genesis where we are told that our primordial ancestors, Adam and Eve, disobeyed God's command not to eat the fruit of a certain tree, and were expelled from the Garden of Eden when they did so. There are four main characters in the story: God, Adam, Eve and the Serpent who tempted Eve to eat the prohibited fruit which she then shared with Adam. Despite the main thrust of this myth, that the disobedience led to the downfall of the human race, the serpent is not castigated as the personification of evil, or given the opprobrious name of Satan or Devil. He/she is merely described as being 'more crafty than any beast of the field that the Lord God had made' and 'accursed more than all cattle and all wild creatures'[14] for tempting the woman.

The acceptance of Satan as the personification of evil probably became part of the Judaic tradition when the Jews were exiled to Babylon in the sixth century BCE and came into close contact with the teachings of Zoroastrianism. Babylon was then the capital of the mighty Persian empire and Zoroastrianism was the state religion. The main feature of this religion was its monotheism, the belief that there was only one God whom they called Ahura Mazda. Zoroastrians also believed that Ahura Mazda had two sons, the twins Spenta Mainyu and Angra Mainyu, and that, at the beginning of time, they had to make a deliberate choice between good and evil. Spenta Mainyu chose goodness whilst Angra Mainyu chose evil and became the personification of evil, the Devil. Other teachings of Zoroastrianism, which the Jews did not hold before their exile, but later came to accept, was a belief in the resurrection of the dead and in a millennium, a new age when creation would be rehabilitated. This wonderful new era would be inaugurated by the appearance of a Messiah who would be the son of a virgin. A major point of disagreement between Jews and Christians has always been whether Jesus of Nazareth was this long awaited Messiah.

Surprisingly, Satan or the Devil figures only occasionally in the Old Testament; while devils in the plural are mentioned on just three occasions. Devils figure much more prominently in the New Testament, where deliverance of people troubled by evil spirits is frequently mentioned in the ministry of Jesus and his disciples. No instances of deliverance are recorded in the Old Testament, though it is full of stories of incest, drunkenness (Noah was the first drunkard), whoring and sacrificing to idols — often common signs, according to some authorities, of demonic possession. Instead, today, the idea is being advanced that possession was averted in Old Testament times by the Mosaic prohibition against communication with the dead, and that this injunction was an effective form of preventive medicine. The expulsion of demons recorded in the New Testament is explained as the active, therapeutic counterpart to the Mosaic prohibition, and a sign that the kingdom of heaven no longer relies only on 'preventive medicine' to deal with demons, but is 'forcefully advancing' against them.[15]

Demonization

An intense preoccupation with demons seems to have been part of the cultural scene in the days of Jesus, and both John the Baptist and Jesus were themselves accused of being possessed[16] or in league with demons.[17] Although the casting out of devils was then an acceptable therapy, it is now of doubtful value and the following incidents indicate where exorcism may have been invoked if the situation had been different.

Example 1: Many years ago, when I was working in a psychiatric unit, an elderly man was admitted to the hospital 'fighting mad'. He had always been physically fit and well-behaved, but there was now a complete change in character that could not be attributed to any medical cause — for instance, a brain tumour. He was a strong, restless person and the nursing staff had considerable difficulty controlling him. It would have been easy to have labelled him as being possessed by demons.

About this time I read of a research project at McGill University which showed that if people are deprived of sensory input, such as sounds or visual images, they can become fearful, hallucinated and irrational. This patient was deaf and had difficulty in understanding what was being said so I examined his ears and found them both full of wax. These were syringed and he regained normal hearing. He also regained his normal pleasant personality and was discharged from hospital, cured.

Example 2: This incident was reported in a medical journal and shows how a person's behaviour can change dramatically and appear demonic. An elderly man called Ernest was admitted to hospital with terminal cancer. His initial behaviour was exemplary but this changed when he learnt the diagnosis and poor outlook, and he soon became 'confused, aggressive, confrontational and obstructive'. The medical staff considered possible explanations, such as hypoxia and opiate analgesia, that might account for his altered behaviour but none was found. Then, in a lucid moment, Ernest asked for a quiet word with one of the junior doctors and told him that he knew his behaviour had changed and it was because he was frightened. He did not mind dying but he was terrified at the idea of being the subject of a postmortem examination and wanted his body to be left alone when he died. The doctor assured him that there would be no postmortem and on hearing that Ernest became his old self again, and one of the nurses' favourite patients. He died two days later.[18]

Example 3: This report also appeared in a medical journal. An army doctor was asked to see an African officer cadet who had been on manoeuvres in the rain-swept hills of Cyprus. The soldier was asserting in a loud muddled voice that he had had a spell cast on him, and kept repeating that his witch doctor had said that he was going to die. A psychiatrist was summoned and whilst they waited for him they took the patient's temperature which was found to be very low, at 32 °C. They gently warmed him up and in two hours he was talking rationally and enquiring in perfect English: 'I don't seem to remember much of the past few hours. Could you let me know what has been happening.' The correct diagnosis was not demonic possession but hypothermia.[19]

We must recognize that there are dangers in believing that we can identify demons, the most crucial being the tendency to project one's own negative propensities on to others. When a group of people, for instance, a nation or a religious body, demonizes any other group then the dangers are magnified. The demonization of the Jews by the Christian Church, which led inexorably to the Holocaust, is evidence of what can happen. This denigration of the Jews became increasingly noticeable over a prolonged period of time. During the first Christian millennium, the relationship between Christians and Jews was not too fraught. Judaism was protected and vilified at the same time, but it was the only belief system among the many ancient religious cults of the Roman empire that Christianity allowed to survive. By the eleventh century, however, attitudes had hardened; Jews were viciously persecuted in France and thousands were massacred in Germany during the First Crusade. This followed a papal declaration that all Jews were guilty for all time of the death of Christ. Later, during the Middle Ages, Jews were depicted for the first time as being in league with the Devil and intent on destroying Christian civilization. Then, during the Age of Enlightenment, their status as human beings was questioned and some groups started to regard them as sub-human. This was the legacy that the Nazis inherited when they decided to purify Europe of all traces of Jewry.[20] The resulting tragedy is well known, but the words of Elie Weisel may help to place it in a more personal context. Of his experiences in a concentration camp he wrote:

> Never shall I forget that night, the first night in camp, which has turned my life into one long night . . . Never shall I forget that smoke . . . the little faces of the children, whose bodies I saw turned into wreaths of smoke beneath a silent blue sky . . . Never shall I forget those moments which murdered my God and my soul and turned my dreams to dust. Never shall I forget those things, even if I am condemned to live as long as God Himself.[21]

Later, on the eve of Rosh Hashanah when the Jews met to mark their New Year festival, surrounded by the electrified wire fence, he felt completely alienated from the scene and from a God who had created Auschwitz, Birkenau and Buna, and who allowed thousands of children to be cremated in his furnaces. He wrote:

> My eyes were open and I was alone, terribly alone in a world without God and without man. Without love or mercy. I had ceased to be anything.[22]

This was the agonizing truth behind the 'Final Solution' and it was not only the Jews who suffered. Other social groups were stigmatized and met a similar terrible fate, among them gypsies, homosexuals and the mentally disabled. Now other sections of the population are being demonized, Freemasons, spiritualists, Hindus[23] and even the bereaved. The following reports give some indication of what is happening in certain churches.

Example 1: Carol looks well but has long-standing physical and emotional problems. She lives alone and manages on a government disability allowance. She has divorced two husbands and her only child died in infancy. There is a past history of attempted suicide and she has received counselling and psychiatric care. Her mother left home when she was a teenager. She is an intelligent woman and a practising Christian who has attended healing services at various churches. Because members of her family have been spiritualists, at one Christian healing centre her problems were attributed to demonic possession and dealt with by deliverance. Her condition remains unchanged and she is constantly looking for new ways to recover a sense of well-being.

Example 2: An elderly Christian lady was terminally ill and diabetic. She attended a Christian healing centre where she was specifically asked if she had been to a Spiritualist church. She admitted to having done so and was informed that she was possessed.

Example 3: A practising Christian applied to join the training course that the Chaplaincy department at her local hospital was running for lay assistants. Her application was rejected because she was a member of the National Federation of Spiritual Healers (NFSH). A bizarre decision as the NFSH is open to people of all ethnic and spiritual backgrounds and many Christians belong to it.

A Note of Caution

As we have already noted, the church authorities distinguish between major and minor exorcisms and say that a major one is rarely required.

They also recognize that this ritual is not without its dangers. The Christian Deliverance Study Group (CDSG) states the position quite clearly:

> Prayer and blessing, the laying-on of hands and/or anointing may be sufficient, and are always appropriate. Exorcism may be positively harmful if it is not the right treatment. It should be used for those cases where non-human malevolent influence is suspected. Human spirits whether incarnate, earthbound or discarnate should not be exorcized. They need, not banishment to hell, but loving care and pastoral concern. When a person is disturbed by the attention of discarnate humans, prayer, blessing and the requiem Eucharist are more appropriate than attempts at banishment.[24]

The emphasis on the loving care of human spirits 'whether incarnate, earthbound or discarnate' is important. As the study group points out, they should not be exorcised, but regretfully it is in this area that Christian healing groups are likely to go astray. They could learn a great deal from the ideas of Dr Kenneth McAll, which are discussed in chapter 6. They could also learn from the Spiritualist Churches whose approach to the troubled bereaved is non-judgemental and is probably quite close to that of the CDSG. There is at present little dialogue between the Christian and Spiritualist churches, but thinking in the latter tends to echo the findings of modern psychiatry that an awareness of the presence of deceased loved ones is perfectly normal and helpful.[25] There is nothing demonic or pathological about such experiences; psychiatrists regard them as part of the normal grieving process and about half of all widowed people will have perceptions of this type. A study at Harvard has looked at the same phenomenon among bereaved children with similar results. It found that most orphaned children continue to be aware of the presence of their dead parent, and the latter often appears to maintain the role of protector or disciplinarian that they had assumed during their lifetime.[26]

The normality of these experiences and the frequency with which they occur is a fairly recent finding and needs to be taken seriously by those responsible for training church workers. It is worth remembering that within a church congregation, half the widowed people will have had experiences of this type and few will have spoken of them to the vicar or minister. It is a very sensitive subject and people still need to be careful in whom they confide this sort of information, as I discovered when I visited a Young Offenders Institution and was asked to see a seventeen-year-old prisoner who had attempted suicide. He had been coping with prison fairly well until he told a 'mate' that his girlfriend, who had recently died in a car crash, was still there with him. When this news became general knowledge he was teased so mercilessly that he attempted to hang himself. Fortunately, he was under close observation and a prison officer was able to rescue him before he asphyxiated. In perceiving the girlfriend, this lad was not evil or possessed, nor was he mentally ill, nor was he consciously trying to establish a renewed relationship with the girl, he was just experiencing one of the common outcomes of bereavement.

Minor Exorcism

The bereaved do not need deliverance or exorcism. They need support, understanding and the assurance that any perceptions they may have that their dead loved one is still with them are perfectly normal. However, sometimes young people get involved in practices which they later come to believe were sinful. These may include consulting astrologers and fortunetellers, and the holding of private seances with Ouija boards or Tarot cards; then they ask for help. Reassurance based on sound common sense may be all that is necessary, but if more is required the Revd Tom Willis recommends the following procedure.[27] He says that the person should be brought to the church altar rail in the presence of at least one priest and, if possible, two other committed Christians. A period of silence and extempore prayer should be followed by a general confession, made by all present, and absolution given. The person then makes a sincere 'Act of Renunciation' by reading from a card the following words.

> In the Name of Jesus Christ, Son of God most High. I [name] renounce the devil and all his works, every occult practice of myself and of my forefathers, and every hold that evil has over me. I commit myself now to the service and protection of Jesus Christ, my Lord and Saviour, who triumphed over evil on the cross, and with the Father and the Holy Spirit, reigns supreme now and forever. Amen

For anyone who wishes to renounce Freemasonry, Tom Willis recommends a similar declaration but which includes the words:

> I [name] renounce my Masonic Oath(s), and I repent of taking part in any idolatrous and blasphemous ritual. I repent of these sins and utterly renounce any evil influence they have brought upon me.

I have attended healing services where people have made similar renunciations, usually standing, and then fallen gently to the floor. At one, I was put under great pressure to renounce my own spiritualist practices, which are non-existent though I have attended services in Spiritualist churches, an experience which enables me to write with some understanding of what happens in them. Most interestingly, the renunciations of the Masonic oath that I witnessed, were not made by Freemasons but by people with relatives who were Freemasons. It seems very odd that individuals should be stigmatized because they are Masons or spiritualists. I have a good deal of sympathy for an elderly Christian who put this question to me recently. 'Why,' he asked, 'should I be made to feel a sinner because I am a Freemason?' For him the accusation must appear even more ludicrous as he worships at a cathedral which was consecrated by a high-ranking Freemason, Bishop Cuthbert Bardsley (Grand Chaplain to the United Grand Lodge of England),[28] and which contains a magnificent stained glass window, a gift of the Freemasons.

A Spiritualist Approach

During the past thirty years I have had occasional contact with the Revd J. Aelwyn Roberts, a priest in the Church in Wales. We first met when the then Archbishop of Wales (Gwilym Owen Williams) asked me to speak to his diocesan clergy on some aspects of bereavement. Since then we have spoken about three times on the telephone. Aelwyn is an octogenarian, now retired, and the author of two books on the afterlife, *Holy Ghostbuster* and *Yesterday's People. A Parson's Search for the Answers to Life after Death*. He does not see a role for exorcism in the care of the 'unquiet dead' and when such problems arise, he turns for help to his Spiritualist friends. Some years ago, he told me the following story and said I could use it in a book. I never thought such an occasion would present itself, but this seems to be an appropriate moment to do so as it illustrates the sort of approach that Spiritualists have to hauntings. I write from memory as I made no notes when I first heard it, though Aelwyn now tells me that it is mentioned in one of his books.

> A woman had been widowed and left with a young family to care for. Her husband had died suddenly and the cause of his death was not clear, but was assumed to be accidental. Later, she found that her nights were being disturbed and this was due to a heaviness on the bed, as if someone was sitting near the foot just as her husband would sometimes do. This happened so often that she felt the need for medical advice and went to see her doctor. Eventually, she was referred to the community psychiatric nurse who spoke to Aelwyn, he visited the lady and then contacted a spiritualist friend who was also a medium. Together, they went to the house and came to the conclusion that the husband was trying to contact the woman and wanted to speak to her. The medium suggested that he would see if the husband would speak to his wife through him, he also suggested that if she would allow herself to be lightly hypnotized she might be able to hear her husband's message at first hand. This idea was accepted by those present. Through the entranced medium the husband informed his wife that he had committed suicide and was dreadfully sorry that he had left her and the children bereft in this way. She was able to discuss the situation with him and express her understanding and forgiveness. This, he said, helped him greatly and he would now be able to proceed to his rightful place in the afterlife.

Spiritualists are not afraid of the dead and do not need the aid of religious symbols when meeting the 'unquiet spirits'. The situation rarely arises, but if asked for assistance they will suggest a psychiatric assessment first and then, if it seems appropriate, an experienced medium will be invited to help. Their methods lack the sense of confrontation implicit in a Christian exorcism. The medium walks though the house, identifies the spirits, reassures them that all is well and encourages them to go to a more suitable place. Their approach seems to be based on direct contact, explanation and persuasion.

Clergy Training

During my career I have been fortunate to meet many members of the clergy of all denominations and have listened to the wide range of views they hold on death, healing and the afterlife. Some, a minority, believe in reincarnation. Most have relatively vague ideas about life after death, while some have lost their faith and no longer believe in an afterlife, which I find very sad. Almost equally poignant is the belief that death is the last enemy to be overcome. I remember the great distress of a young Baptist minister who, though terminally ill, was still striving desperately to stay alive. He was far from reaching the stage of 'acceptance' that Elizabeth Kübler-Ross described even though he had only a few more weeks of earthly life ahead of him.

Christian clergy have an essential role to play when death approaches and during bereavement. Some fulfil this function with great skill and sensitivity, as did the Revd Tom Williams when my parents died, but a substantial number have difficulty with this area of pastoral work and I have occasionally heard people say that they get more support from the undertaker than the clergy. One would expect them to be at ease talking about the significance of death and the hope of resurrection, but it seems to be an area in which they are not particularly well trained and those who become skilful in this field gain their knowledge piecemeal in the years that follow ordination. This personal assessment is confirmed by a report on pastoral care commissioned by the Evangelical Alliance from the University of Wales. Early replies to the questionnaire were from a relatively youthful group. Most (86 per cent) were below the age of 60 and most (80 per cent) had less than twenty years' ministry experience. A surprisingly large number (80 per cent) spoke in tongues, many daily.[29] The report also showed that:

- More than a third (38 per cent) felt they needed further training in the care of the bereaved and dying.

- Few (10 per cent) had regular contact with other professional groups such as doctors, social workers or hospices.
- Most based their pastoral care on common sense (81 per cent) and their own life experiences (89 per cent).
- One fifth (20 per cent) had no formal or recognized training for their pastoral ministry.
- Most (77 per cent) used biblical models of counselling.
- Just 14 per cent used secular models of counselling.
- Almost a quarter (23 per cent) felt they needed more training in how to deal with demonic possession.

That 23 per cent of clergy feel the need for more training in aspects of demonic possession is surprising and points to an almost unhealthy interest in the occult. They also appear to be too isolated from other agencies working with the sick, impoverished and mentally distressed, with only 10 per cent having regular contact with doctors and other professional groups.[30] The opportunities are there to integrate the training of theological students with other disciplines, but when I worked in a hospice that was geographically close to a theological college, we were never invited to talk to the students, even though our education department would have been happy to be involved. On the other hand, we had a close relationship with the Jesuits and their trainees would often spend time, on placement, in the hospice. I think we all benefited from their presence.

A Healing Conference

Healing services and conferences vary greatly in style and intention. Some are quiet, meditative occasions; others are much more proactive. The well-known American evangelist, John Wimber held one at Harrogate and the proceedings were recorded by a social anthropologist, Dr David Lewis, and published in his book *Healing: Fiction, Fantasy or Fact* (1989). The description given was so detailed that some of its findings are worth considering. This was a big conference with 2,470 participants and, of these, just over three-quarters completed questionnaires for Dr Lewis. These showed that over fifty Christian denominations were represented, 8 per cent of participants came from overseas and 129 missionaries and 252 ministers of religion had attended. There were 39 doctors, 133 nurses and 87 workers in other health-related occupations, such as dentistry and radiography. This level of interest indicated the importance of the event and the leader was obviously an attraction as many of those present had been to a previous Wimber conference.

One can deduce from the data given by Lewis that this was a meeting of mainly charismatic and Pentecostal worshippers. Before attending the conference:

- 87 per cent spoke in tongues.
- 55 per cent had words of knowledge.
- 46 per cent could prophesy.
- 42 per cent recognized the presence of spirits.
- 30 per cent interpreted tongues.

These are very high figures and contrast greatly with what one might expect at a medical conference where almost no one would claim to speak in tongues or prophesy or recognize the presence of spirits.

One participant with the gift of discerning spirits described how they manifested themselves. He said that different spirits appear in different forms: perversion appears like a crocodile, a homosexual prostitute, for instance, being described as having a long, greenish snout. Spirits of affliction usually appear as a black lump on the body and I find this interesting as I remember a young man saying that, when he was an alcoholic, he felt that he was carrying a black imp on his shoulder. Demons are sometimes localized on certain parts of the body and their expulsions may be accompanied by physical emissions such as foul odours, deep exhaling, yawning or vomiting.

These signs could be attributed to a withdrawal reaction but, apart from the vomiting, they are not typical of those experienced by drug addicts and alcoholics when being detoxified. The descriptions given above are therefore not in line with normal medical findings, but perhaps the most controversial suggestion made in the report is that a demon can affect not only the body but also the genes.[31]

Being a Christian is apparently no safeguard against possession. This is shown in the relatively high incidence of deliverance practised at the conference where, although most participants were Christians, 6 per cent were treated for demonic possession, women more frequently than men, and younger people (aged below thirty) twice as frequently as those aged over fifty. Their reasons for submitting to the ritual were varied, but essentially they wanted to be delivered from the spirits which they blamed for: transvestism, homosexual activities, masturbation, fear, insomnia, pains in the back; feelings of anger and revenge associated with parental sexual abuse in childhood, and from the linked demons of mockery, sodomy and lust. It was healings following deliverance that were most frequently recorded; there were many fewer physical and inner healings.

Most people attending the conference arrived in good health and any physical ailments they had were relatively minor ones. Within this mainly young and healthy group, 3.6 per cent claimed total healing of a physical condition, a larger number received inner healing whilst, as we have seen, deliverance produced an even higher success rate. A wide range of physical and emotional responses were noted at the conference:

- 52 per cent wept.
- 52 per cent had tingling sensations in the hands.
- 45 per cent reported shaking.
- 44 per cent had changes in breathing.
- 27 per cent said they laughed.
- 19 per cent fell to the ground.
- 11 per cent behaved like drunkards.

These are mostly cathartic responses which, in many instances, the participants had experienced at previous conferences.

Among the charismatic skills practised at the conference were Words of Knowledge. These are thoughts or ideas that come usually intuitively and are interpreted as an indication of an illness or affliction in some other person. Words of Knowledge can also appear as a mental picture or written words or may be linked to a feeling of discomfort in the body. Some practitioners just say whatever comes into their mind. This is not a specifically Christian gift, I have seen Spiritualists and spiritual healers practise it.

The power of a Word of Knowledge is illustrated by a story John Wimber used to tell of seeing the word 'adultery' written on the face of a man whilst they were travelling in an aeroplane. He challenged the man, told him the name of the woman involved and then led him to Christ.[32] Lewis gives other examples of the way John Wimber used Words of Knowledge. He would proceed along these lines, starting with the question:

> What is the patella? It is in the leg — the knee? Is it in the front part or back part? It's in the front? Right, OK. Someone has hurt their patella, the kneecap, and I believe it's in the left leg, and um, I am not sure, I think I am seeing it in reverse and it's the right leg, someone has a painful right knee and the Lord wants to touch you.[33]

I have seen mediums in Spiritualist churches adopt a similar approach, offering wide-ranging suggestions in the expectation that someone present will respond positively to them. One important difference is that mediums work on the assumption that they are in contact with spirit guides whilst charismatic evangelists believe that they are empowered by the Holy Spirit. Both may have had some form of 'peak spiritual experience' which will have reinforced that particular belief. People have approached me in various situations with Words of Knowledge, suggesting that I had a particular problem, usually physical, but the words were never appropriate or meaningful.

One worrying trend in the current climate of deliverance activity is the increasing assertion by some of those involved that Christians — even evangelical and charismatic ones — need deliverance from demonic bondage or evil influences of various kinds. It seems that for them the normal liturgical and sacramental practices of the Church no longer suffice. This attitude is evident in Lewis's writings. He says:

> Those who feel that the frequent diagnosis of demonization among Christians is rather 'over the top' should stop to consider that 55 per cent of my random sample of nurses had been involved in the occult in some form or other, that over a third of the sample reported experiences of the presence of the dead and that other studies have also shown such experiences to be not uncommon.[34]

The Medical Perspective

Most people realize that, over the past two hundred years, doctors have changed their view on the possibility of demonic possession. They no longer believe that the mentally deranged, or troubled, are the victims of evil spiritual forces though they recognize that environmental factors can play a part in the causation of both mental and physical diseases. The close bonds between the doctor, patient and society can also influence the course of an illness and the diagnosis reached. This is particularly so when patients are deemed to be 'possessed' and the frequency with which this label is applied is determined largely by the views of the society in which the patient lives. In rural Greece, for instance, the term *nevra* (nerves) covers a wide range of symptoms and the diagnosis provides a culturally acceptable way of accounting for behaviour that would otherwise be considered unacceptable. It provides a useful explanation for antisocial conduct, which may occur, for instance, when there is conflict within the family or between different generations. When these difficulties cannot be resolved and individuals display the symptoms associated with *nevra*, there is a high probability that, even today, the latter will be attributed to the 'evil eye' or possession by the devil.[35]

A belief in demonic possession remains remarkably strong in some Western countries. An interesting study was undertaken in a Swiss psychiatric clinic of 343 Protestant outpatients who regarded themselves as 'religious'. Of these, one third believed that their illness might have been caused by 'evil spirits' and a similar number had sought release by 'ritual prayers for deliverance' and by exorcism. The prevalence of such attitudes was closely related to church affiliation and, to a lesser extent, the type of illness. Patients attending charismatic churches were most likely to have tried exorcism, particularly if they were suffering from anxiety disorders or schizophrenia. Many felt that the ritual had been helpful, though psychiatrists could find no improvement in their condition. Coercive forms of exorcism actually led to a deterioration in their well-being.[36]

In many parts of the world, diseases such as HIV/AIDS and measles continue to be attributed to evil spirits and this does not help the delivery of effective treatment to the sufferers. In Kenya, where women provide nearly 95 per cent of all health care in rural areas, mothers of the Duruma tribe frequently treat their sick children with an act of exorcism. Like most African peoples, the Duruma believe in the closeness of the spirit world and the mother's ancestral spirits are considered to have a special responsibility for helping to exorcise childhood illnesses.[37]

Every society has its own way of determining when a person is ill and deciding on the particular cause for that illness. The concept of demonic possession was, for many centuries, an acceptable way of accounting for social disorders and the problem of disease, but it has served its purpose and is now more of a hindrance than a help in the management of the emotionally and spiritually distressed. Its possibility still figures largely in the minds of many religious people but, with few exceptions, possession is no longer recognized as a valid diagnosis by psychiatrists or psychotherapists. The extent of this rejection is reflected in a search of the medical press by Sven Desai of the Royal College of General Practitioners.[38] He found that of the millions of indexed papers published in medical journals between 1974 and 2001, only fifty-four dealt in any way with demons, deliverance or exorcism.

Perhaps the last words on this subject should be those of Stephen Parsons, a clergyman and former editor of *Health and Healing*. He writes: 'Of all the belief systems that can potentially harm an individual, the idea that demonic causes lie at the root of many human problems is perhaps the most alarming.'[39] Parsons reminds us that the philosophical thinking behind a diagnosis and choice of treatment should be a matter of critical concern. In the twenty-first century, it is no longer acceptable to ascribe epilepsy or hypomania to demonic forces. After all, we do not continue to bleed patients just because it was once a traditional form of treatment. It was in fact often harmful, particularly to women as they have always been at greater risk than men of becoming anaemic.

The only evidence that deliverance does any good is anecdotal, and the rationale for its practice reinforces a belief in unaccountable demonic forces. This releases individuals from the need to accept responsibility for their own inner turmoil — they can always blame some outside agency — and is in marked contrast to the stance taken by people such as Christian Scientists, who assume total responsibility for their own health and well-being. There is, I think, a place for treatment by catharsis, and if a person insists that he is possessed by a demon, one might usefully exorcise it, but it is not an idea that should be encouraged. Any improvement is likely to be transitory as there is no guarantee that similar beliefs will not arise again. Deliverance should be recognized for what it is, a cathartic type of intervention, provided mainly by amateurs, which is widely performed in many different cultures and is generally known as exorcism.

Finally, I am reminded of a story told of Dr Walter Davies, one of my predecessors in a Welsh country practice. He was asked to see a woman who claimed that she was possessed by a devil. He took her into a room with a centrally placed table and set a lighted candle on it. He then told her to undress and run around the table shouting 'Go away devil, go away devil'. The treatment was surprisingly effective and she never claimed to be possessed by a devil again.

Chapter Eleven
The Drawbacks of Healing

At the end of Chapter 10, we saw how Dr Walter Davies cured a patient in an unconventional way. If he were to try the same treatment in the twenty-first century it would soon be followed by a complaint to the General Medical Council and a charge of professional misconduct. This is one of the hazards associated with medical practice of which doctors are perpetually aware, and which other health care workers are also experiencing with increasing frequency. A natural response to this development is the increasing tendency among doctors to practise 'defensive medicine' and require more X-rays and laboratory tests than are absolutely necessary, just to be on the safe side. Again, the drugs they have at their disposal are far more powerful agents than the herbal remedies of the early 1900s and the side effects can seriously damage patients. When this happens the patient is said to suffer from iatrogenic disease and, if this can be traced to an act of negligence, the doctor is likely to be heavily penalized by both the courts and his/her professional regulatory body.

This scenario is not one that the public associates with the practice of complementary medicine, or of healing *per se*, but all interventions carry an element of risk and this is so despite claims by some therapists that their treatments are totally harmless. This drawback of alternative medicine needs to be mentioned, if only briefly, so that clients can make informed choices when seeking relief. The need to be fully briefed cannot be overemphasized. For instance, before setting out on pilgrimage, particularly to a Third World country, people should make a realistic assessment of their own capabilities and the likely hazards they might meet on the journey so that a happy outcome may result.

Problems for Pilgrims

Pilgrimages can be joyful, social occasions but are rarely without an element of danger and the risk of contracting meningitis during the *hajj* has been mentioned in Chapter 2. Other pilgrim centres present different dangers. On the Indian subcontinent altitude sickness is a real problem for those visiting the holy sites in the Himalayas. A Nepalese doctor who had watched 5,000 people praying to the god Shiva at the mountain lake Gosainkunda in Nepal, wrote: 'I knew that many were in no mood to pray. They were stricken with altitude sickness in its various forms – acute mountain sickness, acute pulmonary oedema, and acute cerebral oedema.'

These are not insignificant indispositions. Acute mountain sickness is relatively benign – it feels like having a hangover with a headache some nausea and tiredness – but it can lead to acute pulmonary oedema and/or acute cerebral oedema, both life-threatening conditions. The situation in Nepal is complicated further because many of the pilgrims observe a fast during their journey eschewing even water and, as a result, become seriously dehydrated. This happens most frequently to the women as they tend to observe the fast more punctiliously than the men.[1]

An increasing number of people from the Western world now visit the Himalayan shrines. These are not predominantly hippies, but devotees who are often elderly and sick. They fly into one of the large cities and then travel swiftly by road to the mountains, allowing themselves little time to acclimatize to the high altitudes. Many are completely unprepared for the harsh conditions they encounter. Not surprisingly, the weakest among them find that the effort needed for the enterprise overwhelms them. They literally fall by the wayside and then have to be rushed to hospital by their fellow travellers disrupting both the pilgrimage and the local health services.

In contrast, pilgrimages to Western shrines, such as Lourdes, are now so well organized that they are really very safe, but one point has been drawn to my attention recently, and that is the possible risk associated with the use of 'holy water' purchased at sites such as Fatima and Lourdes. Bottles of this water are very popular with pilgrims as they make acceptable presents for those at home. The water is perfectly fit for drinking when first purchased; however, once the bottle has been opened the water soon becomes contaminated and can, after a while, cause problems if it is drunk by or even sprinkled on a sick person.

The 'Big Five'

The principal disciplines in complementary and alternative medicine (CAM) are osteopathy, chiropractic, acupuncture, herbal medicine and homeopathy. These are seen as the 'Big Five' by most alternative practitioners and there is an increasing demand for the treatments they offer. The procedures are not entirely without risk and a brief sketch of their more serious complications is appropriate here.

Acupuncture is a relatively safe procedure, but complications can arise and while most are minor some can be life-threatening. In this field under-reporting is likely to be the norm as serious problems may not surface for months. Hepatitis is the most often reported serious complication, but patients have also contracted other potentially lethal infections such as septicaemia and subacute bacterial endocarditis, though the use of properly sterilized needles minimizes the risk of such outcomes. A poor technique can also be a problem and has led to difficulties with pacemakers, cardiac tamponade and pneumothorax. These adverse effects are uncommon but therapists need to be constantly aware of the dangers and so should their clients.[2]

Procedures involving the manipulation of bones and joints can have devastating side effects, which again are very uncommon. Problems are most likely to occur when the neck is manipulated, particularly if the Cl/C2 segment of the cervical vertebrae is involved, as this puts the vertebral artery at risk. Damage at this site may lead to a stroke, usually of the type known as Wallenberg's syndrome, which presents as facial pain, severe vertigo, vomiting, difficulty in swallowing and loss of control of body movements. A survey by the American Academy of Neurology disclosed fifty-five strokes during its two-year study of chiropractic treatment in the United States. Such an outcome is devastating for the patient and practitioner alike but, despite these occasional hazards, a review of the literature confirms that the procedure is still a very safe one.[3] It is the possibility of consequences like these that make it essential for health care workers, whatever their discipline, to be properly trained and insured. Damaged patients are able to seek redress through the courts and the compensation awarded can be very high.

Herbal Medicines

Herbal remedies are currently the most popular segment of the alternative medicine market. Packets of herbs are readily available in shops and pharmacies and most people think they are 'safe' because they are 'natural remedies' and therefore different from mass-produced drugs. This is not necessarily so. Information on the potential toxicity of these remedies is often not well documented or readily available. Because of the risks involved, the United Nations has established a Drug Monitoring Centre (UMC) at Uppsala in Sweden, to collate and analyse the information provided by fifty-five countries which have set up their own drug monitoring and information centres. Unfortunately, India and China have not yet joined this project though they are major users and exporters of herbal remedies.

The first 16,000 adverse reports received by the UMC included twenty-one deaths. Anaphylaxis is the most frequently mentioned critical reaction; others include cases of bronchospasm, circulatory failure and intestinal obstruction. The most frequently incriminated herbal agents are opium alkaloids, evening primrose oil, peppermint oil, psyllium hydrophillic mucilloid, ginkgo tree leaves, mistletoe extract and echinacea extract.[4]

The increasing uptake of herbal remedies poses a particular problem for doctors, a problem that is greater now than when I was in practice. Doctors rarely know when their patients are taking alternative medicines, or following dietary regimes, which are incompatible with the treatments that they are prescribing and this has ceased to be a minor issue but one of growing concern. As an interested observer, I am no longer surprised by the number of people I meet who take alternative medicines in conjunction with those prescribed by their doctor without the latter being aware that this is happening. With homeopathic drugs this probably doesn't matter greatly but when the remedies contain steroids and opioids it can be important.

Asian Herbal Medicines

Chinese herbal medicines (CHM) constitute a multi-billion dollar business. About 500 Chinese medicines are available in the Western market and over 3,000 practitioners offer these remedies in the UK alone. Of the CHM herbs imported into this country, between 10 and 15 per cent are of doubtful authenticity yet there is no control over poor quality or potentially harmful specimens. The problem is being addressed in Europe through the generosity of the Garfield Weston Foundation, which established a Chinese Medicinal Plants Centre at Kew Gardens in London in 1998. This centre works in conjunction with the Institute of Medicinal Plant Development in Beijing to encourage the production of high quality herbs so that greater patient safety is ensured.[5] The need is pressing. Part of the trouble is that herbal remedies are difficult to classify, and this is because they are often a complex mixture of chemicals of uncertain concentrations. The composition of the plant material from which they are derived is determined by many factors, including the weather during growth and the time when they are harvested.[6] There is also much confusion over nomenclature as a wild plant may be known by two or three different names within the same locality. In large countries, where there is a wide variety of languages and dialects, the situation becomes even more uncertain.

Lack of regulations governing the identity and quality of herbs allows adulterated specimens, and plants of dubious origin, to enter the international market. The results for patients can be catastrophic. Some have suffered liver damage, kidney damage and cancer after ingesting medicines obtained from these herbs. Chinese herb nephropathy is a particular problem. This is a rapidly progressive end-stage renal disease, which has occurred most commonly in women who have taken Chinese medicines in their efforts to lose weight. More than a hundred patients have been admitted to hospital in Belgium with this disease and all the cases can be traced to the ingestion of a preparation containing the wrong herbal ingredient, *Aristolochia fangchi*. This plant is not just nephrotoxic; it is also carcinogenic and a high proportion of the women later developed cancer of the ureter or kidney or both.[7]

Some Chinese herbal medicines are known to be useful in the treatment of severe atopic eczema, but there is also evidence that these same medicines can cause liver damage in susceptible individuals. This came to light in a joint report from Amsterdam and London which mentions four such cases and points out that the observed damage does not appear to be dose-related.[8] None of the patients was Chinese, which is interesting in itself as variations in drug metabolism have been reported in people of different ethnic origins. In the UK, banned substances, such as arsenic and mercury, are still to be found in traditional Chinese medicines despite formal warnings to practitioners. The Department of Health is concerned that these medicines may contain other potentially dangerous ingredients.[9]

There is an urgent need for traditional remedies to be regulated with the same stringency as conventional medicines and for the public to be educated in their use. A recent incident involved a student nurse who was admitted to hospital with severe fenfluramine poisoning just two hours after taking her first dose of a Chinese slimming medicine which contained this drug, which works on the central nervous system. Purchasers need to be aware that a Chinese herbal prescription is prepared specifically for them and may contain 10–25 different ingredients from a wide range of plant, animal and mineral material. The fact that the prescription is for a 'herbal remedy' does not automatically mean that it is safe. This point cannot be made too often.[10]

People should take particular care when tempted by on-line therapies. It is now possible to buy medicines advertised on the World Wide Web, and the practice is growing. Not surprisingly there have been reports of serious reactions to the treatments on offer, including two deaths from kidney failure. Although a medicine is advertised on the Web as a herbal remedy, it may contain other ingredients such as steroids, minerals and animal products, and may, in extreme cases, cause serious damage.

Religious Abusers

All professions have black sheep who sully the reputation of their colleagues and who need to be censured by, or even expelled from, their
professional organization. In the UK, disciplinary control of the practice of
osteopathy and chiropractic is now regulated, like that of medicine and
nursing, by Acts of Parliament. The regulating bodies of other CAM therapies are also actively engaged in improving the training and professional
standards of their members, but a recognition of the importance of some
form of control is less apparent in the churches. The only requirement for
the Christian clergy to engage in a ministry of healing is that they have
been commissioned by their bishop (*ipso facto* by Christ) to do so. Most
receive no specific training for this ministry and remain accountable only
to the bishop (or the equivalent authority in a Protestant church), whilst
the bishop is answerable to no one. Lip service is paid to working in conjunction with the medical profession but, apart from hospital chaplaincies,
such co-operation is in practice negligible.

Of the hazards that may be encountered in the search for spiritual healing two are particularly relevant to this chapter. The first is the possibility
of physical abuse by church/spiritual leaders. Stephen Parsons deals with
this in his book *Ungodly Fear*, where he shows how power-oriented leaders
in the Church have harmed individuals seeking their help.[11] This type of
problem did not receive much publicity before the 1990s but the increasing revelations from within the Catholic Church of the way predatory
priests were able to abuse young boys without being apprehended, indicate
the ease with which such behaviour can flourish. This is not a specifically
Christian problem, it is a multi-faith one and abuse is likely to be as common in the mosque, temple or synagogue as in a church. However, the
whole issue has special importance for the Christian healing ministry.
Churches are not always the safe havens people imagine them to be.
Clergy, choirmasters, youth leaders and Sunday school teachers are among
those who have been convicted of sexual abuse yet a high proportion of
these attend church regularly, with 26 per cent of convicted abusers attending church every week compared to 10 per cent of other adults.[12] Churches
are making it more difficult for potential abusers to have easy access to
children in their care, but it is important to remember that adolescents and
vulnerable adults can also suffer physical abuse from the most unlikely people and that, according to Catholic sources, 90 per cent of the victims of
clerical sex abuse are post-pubescent teenage males.[13]

There is also the problem of 'spiritual abuse'. This may take the form of
aggressive preaching or, as David Woodhouse points out, it may occur
when a person is put under pressure to forgive an abuser before their own
inner trauma has been acknowledged and dealt with.[14] They may have feel-

ings of deep-seated anger, anxiety, guilt and shame that need to be resolved before the moment of forgiveness can be reached. This may take a long time. Some people do reach this point fairly quickly and I remember a social worker from Rwanda, who lost all his family in the genocide of the 1990s, saying how he came to realize that he would only gain a measure of peace if he contacted each of the perpetrators, mainly former friends and neighbours, and forgave them. He did this and was healed by the experience. Some people, like this remarkable Rwandan, can respond to personal tragedy in this way, but it should not be expected of everyone. I still meet volunteer workers in Coventry cathedral, who say they cannot forgive the enemy who destroyed their city though they can accept and welcome German visitors.

Misplaced Zeal

Too great an enthusiasm for a particular form of treatment can have unforeseen consequences. Excessive use of laxatives, for instance, can cause dehydration which, in young children, can be a life-threatening condition, yet the practice is still common in some ethnic communities. Similarly, people can go overboard in their enthusiasm for the ministry of healing, a trend that John Gunston noted after he had joined a spiritual community in 1971. About 2,000 people visited the centre each year and so many came for healing that members of the community would spend hours ministering to them. There were many remarkable results but it was mainly people with emotional and spiritual problems who were helped. Only a few with serious physical illnesses gained relief; some were not healed at all. But Gunston was mainly concerned with a darker side to the ministry when he wrote:

> It isn't easy to write like this. With the spread of the ministry of healing in the denominations in recent years, there has been a growth of triumphalism in some quarters – a false triumphalism that regards any suggestion of failure as an indication of faithlessness or hardness of heart.[15]

This is indeed one of the unacceptable aspects of spiritual healing, whether it is practised within or outside the Church. The vulnerable person who is not healed now carries another burden: a sense of failure. They should have more faith. This is not a conclusion medical practitioners would feel happy with, though there are suggestions of it in some branches of alternative medicine. For instance, there is currently a popular belief that if cancer sufferers can adopt a positive attitude to the disease and show a fighting spirit, then their chances of survival are much improved. This would be fine if it were true, though here again the onus is placed firmly on the patient. I can remember the publication of the initial study which supported this viewpoint, but subsequent ones have not replicated its findings. The underlying idea is very attractive, but a comprehensive review of all twenty-seven studies in this field can find little evidence to support the view that psychological coping styles play any part in determining survival rates from cancer.[16]

A healer needs enthusiasm to be effective but enthusiasm can sometimes lead one into forbidden activities. This happened to the Anglican vicar Chris Bain, who established the highly successful 'Nine O'Clock Service' at his church in Sheffield. This started as a charismatic young person's movement, which matured into a personal fiefdom, during which many members of the congregation were manipulated and abused. It ended as a field day for the tabloid press and in Chris Bain's dismissal from his post.[17]

It is, of course, easy to select the occasional, and atypical, example of malpractice, but it should also make us question what the main purpose of the healing service is within the Church today. The answer is perhaps summarized in the opening sentence of *A Time To Heal, A Report for the House of Bishops on the Healing Ministry*, which states: 'The healing ministry is one of the greatest opportunities the Church has today for sharing the Gospel.'[18] This places the Church's approach within an entirely different context from that of other forms of healing, including standard medical and nursing practice, and is a distinction that people should be aware of when they attend church healing services or seek Christian counselling. If I consult a Muslim doctor, I would consider it improper for him to use that opportunity to convert me to Islam, nor did I ever seek to proselytize patients who came to me for medical care. On the other hand, within the context of a Christian healing service, I would expect to invoke the name of Jesus and seek healing through His grace. These appear to be two quite distinct strands within the healing spectrum, but it is possible to unite such polarities by using the Jungian concept of the waterfall which, as he points out, enables two separate streams of water to become contiguous. The uniting factor in healing is inner prayer, the silent prayer one can offer for patients in the surgery is the same silent prayer one offers for people in the quiet moments of a healing service. Moreover, it is a prayer than can transcend different religious affiliations.

Chapter Twelve
Does it Work?

When I commenced my medical studies in 1951, the practice of medicine was very different from the present day. It was less technical and hospital-oriented and far less successful in treating a wide range of acute and chronic disabilities than it is today. But even then, there had been enormous advances in the care provided since the early part of the twentieth century. The maternal mortality rates, for example, had improved dramatically since the 1920s when the likelihood of a woman dying in childbirth was 433 per 100,000 live births in the UK and 689 per 100,000 live births in the United States. Obstetric care has continued to improve and by the year 2000 maternal mortality had fallen to just five deaths per annum.[1] Pregnancy carried real hazards for women seventy years ago and it does still in certain parts of the world, such as Nepal and Somalia, where 1 in 65 women are likely to die as a direct consequence of being pregnant.[2]

One could make a long list of the improvements in medical practice that have transformed health care in the past few decades, but during the same period people have become increasingly eager to seek help from complementary practitioners and spiritual healers of many different traditions. One wonders why this should be so and if the alternative treatments work.

Why Complementary and Alternative Medicine Therapies?

If orthodox medicine is so effective, why do people seek help from other therapists? Research workers say that dissatisfaction with the effectiveness of conventional care is not a major factor; what people do not like is the way it is presented and many have real concerns about the possible side effects of the drugs prescribed for them. Patients also appreciate the amount of time healers allow them for their consultations and cite this as an important reason for choosing complementary medicine, contrasting this with the sense of feeling rushed and unwanted when consulting medical practitioners. Patients are also very pleased with the treatment they receive from CAM therapists and, in addition to any therapeutic benefit, find them very friendly and good communicators. They listen to their problems and are more forthcoming than conventional health care workers with information about the nature and treatment of their complaints. They also appear to be more skilful in the use of active listening techniques and seem genuinely interested in all aspects of their clients' lives.

When I asked a friend about her experience of CAM therapists, she had this to say. Of the reflexologist, I have still got the pain but I always come away from her feeling more relaxed and much better in myself. And of the acupuncturist, he is lovely: he wants to know everything about me, all my problems and everything that has happened to me.

I hear similar comments when people have attended healing services or been treated by a member of the NFSH, and these personal reports give added weight to the findings of a survey on alternative therapies commissioned by the BBC. This showed that 25 per cent of respondents found it helpful, 21 per cent 'just liked it' and 19 per cent 'found it relaxing'.[3] These are very good reasons for visiting a healer and my hairdresser tells me that many women experience similar feelings of relaxation and well-being following a visit to their favourite hairdresser or beautician.

The Efficacy of Prayer

If I had a strangulated hernia or acute glaucoma I would not go to a healer or a priest for help, I would seek the best medical advice available. At the same time I have to accept the evidence, given in Chapter 8, that prayer can, in some mysterious way, help patients with acute coronary thrombosis. So how do we marry these conflicting positions? In my own case, I do so on past experience. Two examples will suffice and I shall try to make them as brief as possible. Both instances occurred when I was working in Mid-Wales.

Case 1: This incident was reported in the *British Medical Journal* in 1968,[4] though I left out one important detail. I was careful not to say that I prayed for the patient, believing that such an admission would be inappropriate in that context. It is a story with two parts, the main events occurring on succeeding Saturdays in the winter of 1963 when main roads in the region were blocked by heavy snowdrifts. One of my partners was ill, and I was scheduled to take five surgeries each Saturday – three morning ones at different locations, one in the afternoon and another in the evening. I was about to start the first surgery when my wife received a call for me to visit an old man at an isolated farmhouse about five miles away. The request was urgent but not one that demanded an immediate visit, so I completed my first surgery and then did the second one in a nearby village. This was about eight miles in the opposite direction from the farm I was to visit. Then the telephone rang again and this time the request to visit was very urgent. I set out immediately and as I travelled, I did two things, I drove as quickly as I could and I prayed that the patient would be alive when I reached the farm. A neighbour opened the gates for me but before we entered the house I knew the man was dead; it was apparent in the face of his nephew as he stood in the farmyard to greet me. It was also apparent in the face of the old man's sister as she sat despondently beside the kitchen fire. I went upstairs alone to the bedroom where a middle-aged woman, his niece, stood quietly gazing at the man's body as he lay on the bed, obviously dead. She told me that he had died just a few minutes earlier so I immediately applied external cardiac massage, then a very new technique, and, to my surprise, within seconds he began to gasp and then to breathe. He was alive but unconscious and the blocked main road prevented us from transferring him to hospital. So we cared for him as best we could at home. By the evening he was regaining consciousness and the next day he was as good as new. We were all delighted by his recovery and, suspecting that he had had a coronary thrombosis, I took a blood sample for the laboratory to test for cardiac enzymes.

His progress was uneventful and the lab report, as I had expected, did indicate a recent coronary thrombosis. The next Saturday was a beautiful day. I did my first two surgeries as previously and again travelled to the farm though this time without any rush or prayer. When I arrived at the farmyard, I knew the man was dead. Nothing was said but exactly the same pattern of events took place as previously, but this time the woman in the bedroom was not the man's niece but the district nurse. He had died a few minutes before I arrived and this time we left him undisturbed. I felt that my prayer had been answered in a very specific way and that the family had been allowed a period of grace in which to prepare themselves for his death, and they had also been spared the distress of a postmortem examination.

Case 2: This incident happened on a Friday morning and began in the local cottage hospital where GPs used to meet Dick Isaac, the visiting surgeon, to discuss any surgical problems with him. There were three of us on this occasion, the surgeon, my old partner and myself. We were talking in matron's office when I suddenly felt that I should not be there and deliberately, though rather self-consciously, offered a silent prayer seeking guidance. I had an instant response; I just knew that I should go to a nearby house, which was occupied by an old lady and her ninety-year-old aunt.

I had never been to the house before and though they were patients of the practice like everyone else in the town, they were on a partner's list. Having tried the experiment of 'seeking guidance', I now had to decide whether to follow it up or ignore it, and feeling very foolish I went to the small terraced house. The front door was open, which surprised me, and there was no answer to my call so I went upstairs and into the bedroom on the right. The single bed was occupied by old lady who was dying and within a few moments of my entering the room she was dead. Shortly afterwards the niece came upstairs having 'just popped to the shops for a few moments'. She was both surprised and pleased to see me. Pleased that I should be present when her aunt had died and surprised that I should be there at all, partly because the old lady though very fragile had seemed perfectly content before she left the house. A few days later she came to me with a gift, the old lady's family Bible.

This incident cannot be described as a healing but there was perhaps a healing element in it and it does show how unexpected the answers to prayer can be. It also underlines some of the ways that general practice has changed in recent decades, as house visits are much more of a rarity nowadays. In contrast, CAM practitioners seem increasingly willing to visit clients in their own homes, and some even take a portable couch with them if this is needed for the treatment.

Reduction of Anxiety

There is growing evidence that healing can reduce feelings of anxiety. This is apparent in many different ways. It surfaces in its most basic form when a patient says to someone, 'I always feel better for just seeing you.' Most healers can probably think of instances when this has happened without their being able to identify any particular reason for the comment being made. It is a compliment one accepts and the elderly beautician I have mentioned previously had this effect, in a most marked way, on patients in the hospice. She would sit alongside them and rub their hands with an emollient cream and they would all feel better for it. None was cured in a physical sense, most of them had terminal cancer, but they did feel better after her visit.

One of the most interesting outcomes of the research undertaken by nurses is the finding that both therapeutic touch (TT) and non-contact therapeutic touch (NCTT) reduce anxiety levels. It does not seem to make any difference whether the therapist makes actual physical contact with the patient or merely holds her hands within their auric field. The crucial factors seem to be the attitude of the nurse towards her patient and the presence of a real intention to heal. If this intention is present, the patient will feel better; if it is absent, no therapeutic benefit is likely to result. There are other forms of hand healing that are very similar to TT (and NCTT) and it is tempting to speculate whether research into them would produce similar findings.

Hand Healing

Hand healing is a recognized technique used by practitioners of TT and Reiki, by spiritual healers, and by ordained clergy in the laying-on of hands. This last practice has the longest pedigree and the others were probably derived from it. In each case, the healer, or blesser, places his/her hands in close proximity to the patient/suppliant with the intention of healing or helping them.

Traditionally, the hands would have been placed firmly upon the head but recently there has been an increasing tendency to place them just within the patient's auric field, a few inches from the skin, in the expectation that, during the procedure, energy will flow from the healer to the one seeking relief. A certain degree of flexibility is permitted whatever method is used, but Reiki practitioners are taught to place their hands directly on their client and in a particular fashion starting at the head and moving down to the feet. In contrast spiritual healers work mainly through the patients' auric fields.

Therapeutic touch was introduced to the American nursing scene in the 1970s and there is probably little difference between this technique and that practised by well-known healers such as Matthew Manning. However, two features distinguish it from other forms of healing. First, it is now established as a recognized nursing tool and one that does not require any religious/spiritual affiliation. Second, it has been subjected to scientific assessment and shown to be an effective nursing aid, most notably in relieving anxiety. This, and the result of an experiment that showed that NCTT could reduce the length of time taken for wounds to heal, are major advances in clinical care. I think that similar findings could probably be obtained from studies into Reiki and spiritual healing as the methods used by the practitioners, and their philosophical approach to healing, are so similar to those of nurses who practise therapeutic touch. The following points of general agreement are found in the three discipines:

- The method can be used by any trained person irrespective of gender, race or religious belief.
- Belief in the effectiveness of the treatment is not needed.
- There is nothing mysterious about the procedure.

- The healing given is part of a natural process, with the healer acting as a channel through which energy flows into the patient reinforcing their immune system so the disease is dealt with at a deep level.[5]

Other interesting points of similarity are:

- The practitioners are mainly women.
- They are 'convergent healers', that is, ordinary people who are not easily distinguished from the rest of society (see Chapter 2).
- They make sure that the patient is comfortably seated, or lying down, before healing is given.

Some of the criteria mentioned above may be found in various Christian healing ministries, but not all. For instance, the comfort of the patient does not appear to be a major consideration at church services, and healing is likely to be given to the elderly sick as they stand or kneel penitentially. The atmosphere on these occasions may be charismatic or quietly contemplative, and the healing rite may be a separate event in itself or incorporated into a mass or eucharist. Whatever the format, the 'laying-on of hands', which may involve anointing with oil, is likely to be a central part of the service. Healing has now become a widespread, though not universal, practice among Christian clergy – it is very uncommon, for instance, in German churches – and those exercising this ministry come from very diverse theological backgrounds. They are, however, most likely to be male and this distinguishes them from the majority of healers outside the Church, who are predominantly women. Their philosophy is also very different as they would not regard 'a healing' as a natural phenomenon but as evidence of divine intervention.

If, as I suggest, the 'laying-on of hands' is fundamentally similar to other modes of 'hand healing' one would expect it to be just as effective. The question arises 'is it more effective?' as some people might claim it to be. Now that nurses have shown that scientific studies are possible in this particular field, a comparison of the effectiveness of the various forms of hand healing seems appropriate and could, and should, be undertaken. This remains true even if one accepts the traditional view that Christian clergy have a moral duty to heal the sick, having been commissioned by Christ, through their bishop, to do so. Such a belief endows the act of healing with a spiritual dimension in which the Christian minister is perceived as a channel, not of a natural energizing force, but of the Holy Spirit and the healing power of Jesus. One wonders if there is any evidence, outside the scriptures, to support this mystical concept.

The Supernatural Element

Objective research is beginning to produce interesting results, but most of the claims made by healers and their clients tend to be anecdotal. In deciding whether to accept these at face value people have to make a fine judgement between being too gullible and too cynical. They also need to remember the long history of charlatanism associated with healing in its many different forms. That said, remarkable things do happen which are not easily explained by the natural sciences and it is important to be open to such a possibility. In doing so one has to question the integrity of the individuals concerned and the accuracy of their observations. I have no problem with the evidence offered for the healing powers of Padre Pio, Dorothy Kerin and Rees Howells and I like, in particular, the sense of total authenticity that Cameron Peddie provides in his description of the vision he had when he first attempted to heal and of the wonderful results of his intervention.

I am particularly fond of healing stories that mention the presence of Christ. One that I found most compelling concerned the Revd Dr Donald English, twice past President of the Methodist Conference, which occurred during his wife's last illness. He spoke of it reluctantly, considering such moments to be too precious to be trumpeted abroad, but refers to the 'signals of divine presence [that] were deeply surprising as well as comforting and challenging' and of twice seeing 'a vision of the risen Christ' when his terminally-ill wife was receiving healing from Esmond Jeffries. Some time after her death, Donald English returned to the bedroom with Jeffries and told him what he had seen there. He described the vision of Christ as being of a solid figure who was present for 3–4 minutes before just walking out through the door. English admitted that if he had heard the story from someone else, he would have questioned its reality. Perhaps most significantly, the wife was not healed but died soon afterwards, yet everyone seemed to have been helped by the ministration of Esmond Jeffries.[6]

Healing has Many Forms

A critical review of this book could point to many approaches to healing that have not been included such as drama therapy, visualization techniques and the contribution that pets can make. Another important field that has been largely unexplored is the area covered by the 'listening therapies', such as the care offered by counsellors and the Samaritans. Many of the practitioners in this field are volunteers and they provide a source of psychological and spiritual support which has enormous importance for the welfare of our modern society.

The ability to listen to, and support, the sick is an essential skill for all healers, but sometimes the sympathetic ear needs to be replaced by the acerbic tongue or at least by unambiguous advice. I still remember an incident that occurred almost forty years ago when we were still doing surgeries on Saturday nights. This was always a trying time at the end of a long working day and one of the last people to enter the room was often an elderly hill farmer. Modern GPs would call him a 'heart-sink' patient, who would stay for ages looking lugubrious and complaining of 'wind around the heart', a local euphemism for angina pectoris. He had had all the tests imaginable, including X-rays and electrocardiograms, and nothing abnormal could be found, but he continued to complain. Eventually, I spoke to him very sharply and said, 'Look, there is nothing wrong with you at all'. He looked very surprised and wanted to know if it was safe for him to walk over the hills, to which I replied of course he could. When he left the surgery he gave me such a look that I thought he would never bother to come again.

I did not see him for some months, and then he reappeared but with a different complaint. The consultation passed by uneventfully then, as he was leaving he turned round and said, 'Do you remember the last time I was here? When you told me there was nothing wrong with me and that I could walk over the hills as much as I wanted?' I said that I did. He continued: 'When I went out through that door, I stopped and thought "what a fool I have been" and you telling me that there was nothing wrong with me, that [and he emphasized the importance of what he was saying by smacking one hand against the other] was the best bottle of medicine I have ever had.' In retrospect it was all so simple, the man had been frightened and needed to be convinced that he could live a normal life and would not drop down dead if he continued to tend his sheep on the mountains.

I have no way of knowing how often cures can be effected in this way but probably not infrequently. A similar incident occurred when I was a junior doctor in a psychiatric hospital and my consultant had admitted a young man with the diagnosis of acute anxiety state. As we chatted I realized that the patient thought he was schizophrenic. I assured him that he was not and told him that there was no need for him to stay in hospital if he did not want to. He immediately picked up his bags and left. Some months later, I was walking along St Mary's Street in Cardiff when I was approached by a very confident and well-dressed man. He had recognized me in the crowd and came to thank me for not admitting him to hospital. It was a very simple act but it was all that was needed to cure the man.

Healing is an emotive subject and everyone must decide for themselves whether it works or not. I believe that it does and that it is most effective in those diseases that are sometimes called psychosomatic, where inner distress manifests itself as a real physical disability. This is not to say that such problems are 'just in the mind'; we know, for instance, that bereavement is associated with an increased mortality among young men[7] and that clinical depression is associated with an increased incidence of physical complaints such as lassitude and backache. Dealing with these diverse morbidities requires insight and a variety of skills including the ability to 'heal'. My farmer was brought to a realization of his self-inflicted limitations by some straight talking. Anxious patients are relieved of their burden by nurses using TT. Spiritual healers are able to help those who are emotionally as well as physically distressed. These are the minor miracles of healing that I can accept wholeheartedly. There are also the reported major miracles such as the healing of Delizia Cirolli mentioned in Chapter 3. These I accept prayerfully, acknowledging with Hamlet 'There are more things in heaven and earth, Horatio, than are dreamt of in your philosophy.'[8]

References

Introduction

1 Kroll U (1991) In Touch with Healing. London: BBC Books, p 3.
2 Carroll L (1871) Through the Looking Glass. Glasgow: Blackie, p 70.

Chapter 1 Who is Dewi Rees?

1 Murray A (1952) Divine Healing. London: Victory Press.
2 Gibbard N (1996) Taught to Serve. The History of Barry and Bryntirion Colleges. Bridgend: Evangelical Press of Wales, p 70.
3 Rees W (1965) Pregnant woman struck by lightning. British Medical Journal 1: 103–4.
4 Rees W (1965) Agricultural tractor accidents. British Medical Journal 2: 63–6.
5 Rees W (1966) Psychotropic drugs and the motorist. The Practitioner 196: 704–6.
6 Rees W (1967) Physical and mental disabilities of 1,190 ordinary motorists. British Medical Journal 1: 593–7.
7 Rees W, Lutkins S (1967) Mortality of bereavement. British Medical Journal 4: 13–16.
8 Rees W (1968) The immediate care of road traffic and tractor accidents in a rural community. Journal of the Royal College of General Practitioners 15: 115–22.
9 Rees W, Lutkins S (1971) Parental depression before and afterchildbirth. Journal of the Royal College of General Practitioners 21: 26–31.
10 Rees W (1971) The hallucinations of widowhood. British Medical Journal 4: 37–41.
11 Rees W, Jenkins H (1972) Pulmonary embolus. British Medical Journal 2: 102.
12 Rees W (1972) The distress of dying. British Medical Journal 3: 105–7.

Chapter 2 Healing in Different Cultures

1   Gottlieb S (2000) UN says up to half of the teenagers in Africa will die of AIDs. British Medical Journal 321: 67.

2   Lee K (2001) Healing the African way. Healing Today 84: 9–10.

3   Mbiti J (1969) African Religions and Philosophy. London: Heinemann, p 20.

4   Devisch R (1985) Polluting and healing among the Northern Yaka of Zaire. Social Science and Medicine 21(6): 693–700.

5   Devisch R (1985) Polluting and healing among the Northern Yaka of Zaire. Social Science and Medicine 21(6): 693–700.

6   Cepe M (1997) Cultural issues in Filipino healing. In G Calvert (Ed) Health, Healing and Wholeness. London. The Salvation Army, pp 153–4.

7   Koss J (1986) Expectations and outcomes for patients given mental health care or spiritualist healings in Puerto Rico. American Journal of Psychiatry 144(1): 56–61.

8   Silverblatt I (1983) The evolution of witchcraft and the meaning of healing in colonial Andean society. Culture, Medicine and Psychiatry 7: 413–27.

9   Gibbins R (1943) Coming down the Wye. Books Inc. Distributed by EP Dutton, New York, p 9.

10 Morris J (1888) The Art of Talismanic Magic. Being selections from the works of Rabbi Solomon, Agrippa, Barrett etc. Manuscript department of the National Library of Wales, Aberystwyth. Code number NLW, manuscript 11297C.

11 Gibbins R (1943) Coming down the Wye. Books Inc. Distributed by EP Dutton, New York, pp 129–30.

12 Kerewsky-Halpern B (1985) Trust, talk and touch in Balkan folk healing. Social Science and Medicine 21(3): 319–25.

13 Appleby C (2001) Ayurvedic Therapy – A Personal Experience. Towards Wholeness. No. 101. Friends Fellowship of Healing.

14 Kapur R (1979) The role of traditional healers in mental health care in rural India. Social Science and Medicine 13B: 27–31.

15 Salan R, Maretzki T (1983) Mental health services and traditional healing in Indonesia: are the roles compatible? Culture, Medicine and Psychiatry 7: 377–412.

16 Salan R, Maretzki T (1983) Mental health services and traditional healing in Indonesia: are the roles compatible? Culture, Medicine and Psychiatry 7: 377–412.

17 Salan R, Maretzki T (1983) Mental health services and traditional healing in Indonesia: are the roles compatible? Culture, Medicine and Psychiatry 7: 377–412.

18 Constantinides P (1985) Women heal women: spirit possession and segregation in a Muslim society. Social Science and Medicine 21(6): 685–6.

19 Constantinides P (1985) Women heal women: spirit possession and segregation in a Muslim society. Social Science and Medicine 21(6): 690–1.

20 New English Bible (1972) Genesis 17: 10–14.

21 Szabo R, Short R (2000) How does male circumcision protect against HIV infection? British Medical Journal 320: 1592–94.

22 Davies G (1963) Deuteronomy. In Matthew Black and HH Rowley (Eds) Peake's Commentary on the Bible. London: Thomas Nelson, pp 276–7.

Chapter 3 Pilgrimages and their Healing Role

1   Farmer D (1997) The Oxford Dictionary of Saints. Oxford and New York: Oxford University Press, p 54.
2   Dahlberg A (1991) The body as a principle of holism: three pilgrimages to Lourdes. In J Eade and MJ Sallnow (Eds) Contesting the Sacred. The Anthropology of Christian Pilgrimage. London: Routledge, p 35.
3   Dahlberg A (1991) The body as a principle of holism: three pilgrimages to Lourdes. In J Eade and MJ Sallnow (Eds) Contesting the Sacred. The Anthropology of Christian Pilgrimage. London: Routledge, p 37.
4   Billet B and Lafourcade P (1981) Lourdes Pélérinage. (Eade's translation). Paris: de Brouwer, p 170.
5   Dahlberg A (1991) The body as a principle of holism: three pilgrimages to Lourdes. In J Eade and MJ Sallnow (Eds) Contesting the Sacred: The Anthropology of Christian Pilgrimage. London: Routledge, p 43.
6   Dahlberg A (1991) The body as a principle of holism: three pilgrimages to Lourdes. In J Eade and MJ Sallnow (Eds) Contesting the Sacred: The Anthropology of Christian Pilgrimage. London: Routledge, p 45.
7   Eade J (1991) Order and power at Lourdes. Lay helpers and the organisations of a pilgrimage shrine. In J Eade and MJ Sallnow (Eds) Contesting the Sacred. The Anthropology of Christian Pilarimage. London: Routledge, pp 55–63.
8   Dulake M (2000) personal communication.
9   Eade J (1991) Order and power at Lourdes. In J Eade and MJ Sallnow (Eds) Contesting the Sacred. The Anthropology of Christian Pilgrimage. London: Routledge, p 72.
10 Dowling S (1984) Lourdes cures and their medical assessment. Journal of the Royal Society of Medicine 77: 635–6.
11 Dowling S (1984) Lourdes cures and their medical assessment. Journal of the Royal Society of Medicine 77: 637.
12 Dowling S (1984) Lourdes cures and their medical assessment. Journal of the Royal Society of Medicine 77: 636.
13 Morris P (1982) The effect of pilgrimage on anxiety, depression and religious attitude. Psychological Medicine 12: 291–4.
14 McKevitt C (1991) San Giovanni Rotondo and the shrine of Padre Pio. In J Eade and MJ Sallnow (Eds) Contesting the Sacred. The Anthropology of Christian Pilgrimage. London: Routledge, pp 77–97.
15 McCaffery J (1978) The Friar of Giovanni. Tales of Padre Pio. London: Darton, Longman and Todd.
16 Bowman G (1991) Christian ideology and the image of the holy land: the place of Jerusalem pilgrimage in the various Christianities. In J Eade and MJ Sallnow (Eds) Contesting the Sacred. The Anthropology of Christian Pilgrimage. London: Routledge, p 112.

17   Bowman G (1991) Christian ideology and the image of the holy land: the place
     of Jerusalem pilgrimage in the various Christianities. In J Eade and MJ Sallnow
     (Eds) Contesting the Sacred. The Anthropology of Christian Pilgrimage.
     London: Routledge, p 120.
18   Stirrat R (1991) Place and person in Sinhala Catholic pilgrimage. In J Eade and
     MJ Sallnow (Eds) Contesting the Sacred. The Anthropology of Christian
     Pilgrimage. London: Routledge, pp 132–3.
19   Stirrat R (1991) Place and person in Sinhala Catholic pilgrimage. In J Eade and
     MJ Sallnow (Eds) Contesting the Sacred. The Anthropology of Christian
     Pilgrimage. London: Routledge, p 126.
20   Stirrat R (1991) Place and person in Sinhala Catholic pilgrimage. In J Eade and
     MJ Sallnow (Eds) Contesting the Sacred. The Anthropology of Christian
     Pilgrimage. London: Routledge, pp 133–4.
21   Sanwar G (1996) Islam: a Brief Guide. London: The Muslim Educational Trust.
22   Salloum H (1998) Following the steps of Saint Paul in Damascus. World Faiths
     Encounter. 20: 46–9.
23   The Holy Qur'ān. Text, Translation and Commentary by Abdullah Yūsuf Alī
     (1989) Maryland: Amana Corporation, Sūrah 12, pp 574–8.
24   Gatrad A, Sheikh A, Khan A (2002) Reducing health risk to Muslim pilgrims.
     British Medical Journal (Letters) 324: 301.
25   Dynes M (2000) Black magic cave fuels white resentment. The Times. Friday, 4
     August, p 19.
26   Reed A (1999) Help the Poorest on Earth. A newsletter from Ethiopiaid.

Chapter 4 Judaeo-Christian Perspective

1   Botting M (1998) Christian Healing in the Parish. Nottingham: Grove Books,
     pp 6–8.
2   The New English Bible (1979) Genesis 20: 17–18.
3   Neil W (1962) William Neil's One Volume Bible Commentary. London.
     Hodder and Stoughton, pp 125–6.
4   New English Bible (1979) 1 Kings 17: 19–22.
5   New English Bible (1979) 2 Kings 4: 28–35.
6   Rees W (1968) Personal view. British Medical Journal 1: 701.
7   New English Bible (1979) 2 Kings 4: 38–41.
8   New English Bible (1979) 2 Kings 5: 1–14.
9   Waterson A (1962) Disease and healing. In The New Bible Dictionary. p 316.
     Quoted by Botting, M (1998) Christian Healing in the Parish. Nottingham:
     Grove Books, p 8.
10   Botting M (1998) Christian Healing in the Parish. Nottingham: Grove Books.
11   New English Bible (1979) Acts 5: 15–16.
12   New English Bible (1979) Acts 28: 8–9.
13   New English Bible (1979) 1 Philippians 2: 25–30.
14   New English Bible (1979) 2 Timothy 4: 20.

15 New English Bible (1979) 1 Timothy 5: 23.

16 New English Bible (1979) James 5: 13–16.

17 Bennetts Bishop Colin (2000) Service for the Ordination of Deacons and Priests at Coventry Cathedral. July 2nd.

18 Amundsen D, Ferngren G (1988) The Early Christian Tradition. In RL Numbers and D Amundsen (Eds) Caring and Curing: Health and Medicine in Western Religious Traditions. Baltimore: Johns Hopkins University Press, pp 48–9.

19 Amundsen D, Ferngren G (1988) The Early Christian Tradition. In RL Numbers and D Amundsen (Eds) Caring and Curing: Health and Medicine in Western Religious Traditions. Baltimore: Johns Hopkins University Press, p 52.

20 Gardner R (1983) Miracles of healing in Anglo-Celtic Northumbria as recorded by the Venerable Bede and his contemporaries; a reappraisal in the light of twentieth-century experience. British Medical Journal 287: 1927–33.

21 Farmer D (1997) The Oxford Dictionary of Saints. Oxford: Oxford University Press, p 45.

22 Amundsen D (1988) The medieval Catholic tradition. In RL Numbers and D Amundsen (Eds) Caring and Curing: Health and Medicine in Western Religious Traditions. Baltimore. Johns Hopkins University Press, p 98.

23 Castle E, Kennedy C (1980) St Mary's, St Osburg's and All the Saints. Coventry City Council Archivist Department. Coventry through Time. Booklet 3.

24 New English Bible (1979) Acts 19: 11–12.

25 Amundsen, D (1988) The medieval Catholic tradition. In RL Numbers and D Amundsen (Eds) Caring and Curing: Health and Medicine in Western Religious Traditions. Baltimore: Johns Hopkins University Press, p 71.

26 Davies E (1999) Concerning Cults. Evangelical Times. September, p 27.

27 Larner C (1984) Witchcraft and Religions. Oxford: Basil Blackwell.

28 Eyre K (1974) Witchcraft in Lancashire. Lancaster. Dalesman Books, pp 52–3.

29 Moynagh P (2002) Keeping tabs on the Royal Touch. The Times (Letters) 28 May, p 19.

30 Cadbury H (1948) George Fox's Book of Miracles. Cambridge: Cambridge University Press.

31 Hodges D (1995) George Fox and the Healing Ministry. Guildford. Friends Fellowship of Healing, pp 8 and 28–30.

32 Walsh K et al (2002) Spiritual beliefs may affect outcome of bereavement: prospective study. British Medical Journal 324: 1551–4.

33 Hodges D (1995) George Fox and the Healing Ministry. Guildford: Friends Fellowship of Healing, pp 28–30.

Chapter 5 Healing: The Field Widens

1   Booty J (1986) The Anglican tradition. In RL Numbers and D Amundsen (Eds) Caring and Curing: Health and Medicine in the Western Religious Traditions. Baltimore: Johns Hopkins University Press, p 241.

2   Vanderpool H (1998) The Wesleyan-Methodist tradition. In RL Numbers and
    D Amundsen (Eds) Caring and Curing: Health and Medicine in the Western
    Religious Traditions. Baltimore: Johns Hopkins University Press, p 329.
3   Congreve W (1685) Love for Love. 2: 5.
4   Wardle J (2001) Music and healing. Acorn, the Magazine of the Acorn
    Christian Foundation. Issue 8, pp 5–6.
5   Vickers A, Zollman C (2000) ABC of complementary medicines: Homeopathy.
    British Medical Journal 319: 1115–18.
6   Bush L (1998) The Mormon tradition. In RL Numbers and D Amundsen (Eds)
    Caring and Curing: Health and Medicine in the Western Religious Traditions.
    Baltimore: Johns Hopkins University Press, p 403.
7   Bush L (1998) The Mormon tradition. In RL Numbers and D Amundsen (Eds)
    Caring and Curing: Health and Medicine in the Western Religious Traditions.
    Baltimore: Johns Hopkins University Press, p 404.
8   Bush L (1998) The Mormon tradition. In RL Numbers and D Amundsen (Eds)
    Caring and Curing: Health and Medicine in the Western Religious Traditions.
    Baltimore: Johns Hopkins University Press, pp 403–4.
9   Schoepflin R (1986) The Christian Science tradition. In RL Numbers and D
    Amundsen (Editors) Caring and Curing: Health and Medicine in the Western
    Religious Traditions. Baltimore: Johns Hopkins University Press, pp 429–30.
10 Harper T (1994) The Uncommon Touch. An Investigation of Spiritual
    Healing. Toronto: McClelland and Stewart, p 45.
11 Peel R (1987) Spiritual Healing in a Scientific Age. San Francisco: Harper and
    Row, p 19.
12 Eddy M (1925) Church Manual of the First Church of Christ Scientist, in
    Boston, Massachusetts, 89th edition. p 15.
13 Eddy M (1925) Church Manual of the First Church of Christ Scientist, in
    Boston, Massachusetts, 89th edition. p 16.
14 Scharwz T (1993) Healing in the Name of God. Grand Rapids: Michigan.
    Zondervan Publishing House, p 128.
15 Peel, R (1987) Spiritual Healing in a Scientific Age. San Francisco: Harper and
    Row, pp 154–6.
16 Bishop M (2002) Should doctors be the judges of medical orthodoxy? The
    Barker case of 1920. Journal of the Royal Society of Medicine 95: pp 41–5.
17 Andrews E, Courtenay A (1999) The Essentials of McTimoney Chiropractic.
    London. Thornsons, pp 48–51.
18 Hocken P (1997) Streams of Renewal (revised edition). Cumbria: Paternoster
    Press, p 1.
19 Jones B (1995) Voices from the Welsh Revival 1904–1905. Bridgend:
    Evangelical Press of Wales, p 26.
20 Wacker G (1998) The Pentecostal tradition. In RL Numbers and D Amundsen
    (Eds) Caring and Curing: Health and Medicine in the Western Religious
    Traditions. Baltimore: Johns Hopkins University Press, pp 514–21.
21 Latham D (1997) A Faith that Works. Bristol: Terra Nova Publications, p 72.
22 Ness R (1980) The impact of indigenous healing activity: an empirical study of
    two fundamentalist churches. Social Science and Medicine 14B: 167–80.

23 Hocken P (1997) Streams of Renewal (revised edition). Cumbria: Paternoster Press, p 140.
24 The Tablet (2001) Charismatics quiz Roman curia over healing document. 24 November. pp 1684–5.

Chapter 6 Spiritual Healers (Christian)

1   Grubb N (1981) Rees Howells Intercessor (seventh impression). Guildford and London: Lutterworth Press.
2   Grubb N (1981) Rees Howells Intercessor (seventh impression). Guildford and London: Lutterworth Press, p 237
3   Grubb N (1981) Rees Howells Intercessor (seventh impression). Guildford and London: Lutterworth Press, pp 90 and 103.
4   Grubb N (1981) Rees Howells Intercessor (seventh impression). Guildford and London: Lutterworth Press, pp 178–81.
5   Peddie J (1966) The Forgotten Talent. London: Fontana, p 28.
6   Peddie J (1966) The Forgotten Talent. London: Fontana, pp 15–16.
7   Peddie J (1966) The Forgotten Talent. London: Fontana, p 49.
8   Peddie J (1966) The Forgotten Talent. London: Fontana, pp 148–51.
9   Ernest J (1987) Dorothy Kerin. Oxford: University Printing House, p 29.
10 Bardsley C (1974) Foreword to Kathleen Browning, See Through. Quoted in Ernest J (1987) Dorothy Kerin. Oxford: University Printing House, pp 74–5.
11 Kerin D (1914) The Living Touch. Obtainable from the Dorothy Kerin Trust, pp 8–13. Quoted in M Maddocks (1999) The Vision of Dorothy Kerin. Guildford: Eagle, pp 12–14.
12 Maddocks M (1999) The Vision of Dorothy Kerin. Guildford: Eagle, p 280.
13 Maddocks, M (1999) The Vision of Dorothy Kerin. Guildford: Eagle, p 281.
14 Arnold D (1965) Dorothy Kerin: Called by Christ to Heal. London: Hodder and Stoughton, pp 49–50. Quoted in Maddocks M (1999) The Vision of Dorothy Kerin. Guildford: Eagle, pp 22–6.
15 Maddocks M (1999) The Vision of Dorothy Kerin. Guildford: Eagle, pp 68–76.
16 Maddocks, M (1999) The Vision of Dorothy Kerin. Guildford: Eagle, pp 60–4.
17 Burrswood (2000) Our History. Leaflet obtainable from Burrswood, Groombridge, Kent, TN3 9PY.
18 Maddocks M (1999) The Vision of Dorothy Kerin. Guildford: Eagle, pp 208–9.
19 Fisher E (1993) Healing Miracles. London: Fount, p 75.
20 New English Bible (1979) James 5: 14.
21 Peddie J (1966) The Forgotten Talent. London: Fontana, p 82.
22 MacNutt F (1974) Healing. Indiana: Ave Maria Press, p 13.
23 Sanford A (1972) Sealed Orders. New Jersey: Logos International, p 99.
24 Sanford A (1972) Sealed Orders. New Jersey: Logos International, pp 107–11.
25 Clark G (1949) Introduction to A Sanford, The Healing Light. London: Arthur James.
26 Sanford A (1949) The Healing Light. London: Arthur James, pp viii–ix.

27 Booty J (1986) The Anglican Tradition. In RL Numbers and D Amundsen (Eds) Caring and Curing: Health and Medicine in the Western Religious Traditions. Baltimore: Johns Hopkins University Press, pp 256–7.

28 McAll K (1982) Healing the Family Tree. London: Sheldon, p 2.

29 McAll K (1982) Healing the Family Tree. London: Sheldon, p 88.

30 McAll F (1996) Family Tree Ministry Journal, p 3.

31 McAll F (1982) Healing the Family Tree, London: Sheldon, pp 22–34.

32 McAll F (1982) Healing the Family Tree. London: Sheldon, p 121.

33 Moll C (1992) Reflections ... a letter to Dr McAll. Newsletter 7. Family Tree Ministry. Summer 1992: p 6.

34 Harrell D (1985) Oral Roberts and American Life. Bloomington: Indiana University Press. pp vii–viii.

35 Sproull O (1954) Preface to Oral Roberts, If you Need Healing Do These Things. Oklahoma: Healing Waters Inc.

36 Harrell D (1986) The Disciples of Christ-Church of Christ Tradition. In RL Numbers and D Amundsen (Eds) Caring and Curing: Health and Medicine in the Western Religious Tradition. Baltimore: Johns Hopkins University Press, p. 391.

37 Harpur T (1994) The Uncommon Touch. An Investigation of Spiritual Healing. Toronto: McClelland and Stewart, pp 28–30.

38 Wacker G (1986) The Pentecostal Tradition. In RL Numbers and D Amundsen (Eds) Caring and Curing: Health and Medicine in the Western Religious Traditions. Baltimore: Johns Hopkins University Press, pp 528–31.

39 Wacker G (1986) The Pentecostal Tradition. In RL Numbers and D Amundsen (Eds) Caring and Curing: Health and Medicine in the Western Religious Traditions. Baltimore: Johns Hopkins University Press, p 531.

40 Harpur T (1994) The Uncommon Touch. An Investigation of Spiritual Healing. Toronto: McClelland and Stewart.

41 Roberts O (1954) If You Need Healing Do These Things.Oklahoma: Healing Water Inc. p 42.

Chapter 7 Other Famous Healers

1 CHO (1997) Leaflet issued by the Confederation of Healing Organizations.

2 CHO (1989) Confederation of Healing Organizations Code of Conduct. Published by the SNU Guild of Spiritualist Healers. July 1989. Guild Office. Keighley, West Yorkshire.

3 New English Bible (1979) Luke 11: 14–20.

4 NU (1999) Pocket Guide to Spiritualism. Essex: Spiritualist National Union Publications.

5 Hawkins J (2000) Healing Today (Letters): November. No. 86, p 33.

6 Barbanell M (1982) In Ramus Branch, Harry Edwards: The Life Story of the Great Healer. Guildford: Burrows Lea, p 7.

7   Branch, R, Harry Edwards: The Life Story of the Great Healer. Guildford: Burrows Lea, pp 71–2.
8   Branch, R, Harry Edwards: The Life Story of the Great Healer, Guildford: Burrows Lea, p 94.
9   Branch, R, Harry Edwards: The Life Story of the Great Healer, Guildford: Burrows Lea, pp 121–2.
10   Branch, R, Harry Edwards: The Life Story of the Great Healer, Guildford: Burrows Lea, p 176.
11   Branch, R, Harry Edwards: The Life Story of the Great Healer, Guildford: Burrows Lea, pp 253–61.
12   Hutton J (1978) Healing Hands (second edition). London: WH Allen, pp 32–5.
13   Gilling L (1986) Bright Shines the Sunlight. London and New York: Regency Press, p 155.
14   Gilling L (1986) Bright Shines the Sunlight. London and New York: Regency Press, p 156.
15   Hutton, J (!978) Healing Hands (second edition). London: WH Allen, pp 14–23.
16   Hutton J (1978) Healing Hands (second edition). London: WH Allen, pp 37–8.
17   Bro H (1990) Edgar Cayce. A Seer out of Season. Wellingborough: The Aquarian Press, pp 52–3.
18   Bro H (1990) Edgar Cayce. A Seer out of Season. Wellingborough: The Aquarian Press, pp 235–7.
19   Bro H (1990) Edgar Cayce. A Seer out of Season. Wellingborough: The Aquarian Press, pp 244–5.
20   Bro H (1990) Edgar Cayce. A Seer out of Season. Wellingborough: The Aquarian Press, p 285.
21   Cayce E (1943) Edgar Cayce. His Life and Work. Booklet, p 10.
22   Bro, H (1990) Edgar Cayce: A Seer out of Season. Wellingborough: The Aquarian Press, p 119.
23   Bro H (1990) Edgar Cayce. A Seer out of Season. Wellingborough: The Aquarian Press, p 94.
24   Mitchell P, Furomoto P (1985) The Usui Gift of Natural Healing. Idaho: The Reiki Alliance.
25   Shuffrey S (2000) Reiki. London: Teach Yourself Books/Hodder and Stoughton, pp 13–15.
26   Kumar K, Hovgaard J (1995) Sai Baba. Source of Light, Love and Bliss. New Delhi: Sterling Paperbacks, p 100.
27   Kennedy D (2001) Three died after putting their faith in guru. The Times. Monday, 27 August, p 3.
28   Manikal M (2000) A memorable patient. The power of prayer. British Medical Journal 321: 550.
29   Kumar, K, Hovgaard, J (1995) Sai Baba. Source of Light, Love and Bliss. New Delhi: Sterling Paperbacks, pp 19–21.
30   Manikal, M (2000) A memorable patient. The power of prayer. British Medical Journal 321: 550.
31   MacDonnell M (1999) Alexander Technique. London: Lorenz Books, p 9.

32 Ball S (1999) The Bach Flower Gardener. Saffron Walden: CW Daniel, pp 40–1.
33 Bach E (1934) The Twelve Healers and Other Remedies. Saffron Walden: CW Daniel, p 5.
34 Viagas B (1997) Pocket A–Z of Natural Healthcare. Dublin: Newleaf, pp 101–2.
35 Apple DJ (1999) Editorial on Sir Harold Ridley. Archives of Ophthalmology 120: 1198.

Chapter 8 Scientific Studies on Healing

1   Morris J (1888) The Art of Talismanic Magic. Being Selections from the Works of Rabbi Solomon, Agrippa, Barrett etc. Manuscript Department of the National Library of Wales, Aberystwyth. Code number NLW, manuscript 11297C.
2   Hodges R, Scofield A (1995) Is spiritual healing a valid and effective therapy? Journal of the Royal Society of Medicine 88: 203–7.
3   Benor D (1993) Healing Research, Holistic Energy Medicine and Spirituality. Volume 1. Deddington: Helix.
4   Bunnell T (1999) The effect of 'healing with intent' on pepsin enzyme activity. Journal of Scientific Exploration (2): 139–42.
5   Nash C (1982) Psychokinetic control of bacterial growth. Journal of the Society for Psychical Research 51: 217–21.
6   Scofield T, Hodges D (1991) Demonstration of a healing effect in the laboratory using a simple plant model. Journal of the Society for Psychical Research 57: 321–43.
7   Benor, D (1993) Healing Research. Holistic Energy Medicine and Spirituality. Volume 1. Deddington: Helix, p 182.
8   Grad B, Cadoret R, Paul G (1961) The influence of an unorthodox method of treatment on wound healing in mice. International Journal of Parapsychology 3: 5–24.
9   Grad B (1965) Some biological effects of laying-on of hands: A review of experiments with animals and plants. Journal of the American Society for Psychical Research 59: 95–112.
10 Sayre-Adams J. Wright S (2001) Therapeutic Touch (second edition). London. Harcourt, p 32.
11 Benor, D (1993) Healing Research. Holistic Energy Medicine and Spirituality. Volume 1. Deddington: Helix.
12 Krieger D (1975) Therapeutic touch: The imprimatur of nursing. American Journal of Nursing 7: 784–7.
13 Heidt P (1981) Effects of therapeutic touch on the anxiety level of hospitalized patients. Nursing Research 30: 30–7.
14 Ferguson C (1986) Subjective Experience of Therapeutic Touch Survey (SETTS): Psychometric Examination of an Instrument (Doctoral dissertation, University of Texas at Austin). Quoted by Benor, D (1993) Healing Research. Holistic Energy Medicine and Spirituality. Volume 1. Deddington: Helix, pp 235–7.

15 Quinn J (1982) An Investigation of the Effect of Therapeutic Touch without Physical Contact on State Anxiety of Hospitalized Patients (Doctoral dissertation, New York University 1982). Quoted by Benor, D (1993) Healing Research, Holistic Energy Medicine and Spirituality. Volume 1. Deddington: Helix, pp 232–4.

16 Fedoruk R (1984) Transfer of the Relaxation Response: Therapeutic Touch as a Method for Reduction of Stress in Premature Neonates (Doctoral dissertation, University of Maryland). Quoted by Benor, D (1993) Healing Research. Holistic Energy Medicine and Spirituality. Volume 1. Deddington: Helix Healing Research, p 238.

17 Wirth D (1989,1990) Unorthodox healing: The effect of noncontact therapeutic touch on the healing rate of full thickness dermal wounds (MA thesis, JFK University). Summarized in L Henkel and J Palmer (Eds) 1989 Research in Parapsychology 190: 47(52. Also in Wirth D (1990) Subtle Energies 1(l): 1–20.

18 Brown C (1995) Spiritual healing in general practice using a quality of life questionnaire to measure outcome. Complementary Therapies in Medicine 3: 230–3.

19 Dixon M (1998) Does 'healing' benefit patients with chronic symptoms? A quasi-randomized trial in general practice. Journal of the Royal Society of Medicine 91: 183–8.

20 Miller R (1982) Study on the effectiveness of remote healing. Medical Hypotheses 8: 481–90.

21 Beutler J, Attevelt J et al (1988) Paranormal healing and hypertension. British Medical Journal 296: 1491–4.

22 Attevelt J (1988) Research into Paranormal Healing (Doctoral dissertation, State University of Utrecht). Quoted by Benor, D (1993) Healing Research. Holistic Energy Medicine and Spirituality. Volume 1. Deddington: Helix Healing Research. pp 218–20.

23 Galton F (1872) Statistical enquiries into the efficacy of prayer. Fortnightly Review 12: 125–35.

24 Joyce C, Welldom R (1965) The efficacy of prayer: A double blind clinical trial. Journal of Chronic Diseases 18: 367–77.

25 Collip P (1969) The efficacy of prayer: A triple-blind study. Medical Times 97(5): 201–4.

26 Byrd R (1988) Positive therapeutic effects of intercessory prayer in a coronary care population. Southern Medical Journal 81(7): 826–9.

27 Sloan R, Bagiella E, Powell T (1999) Religion, spirituality and medicine. The Lancet 353: 664–7.

28 Harris W, Gowda M, Kolb J et al (1999) A randomized, controlled trial of the effects of remote, intercessory prayer on outcomes in patients admitted to the coronary care unit. Archives of Internal Medicine 159(19): 2273–6.

29 Harris W, Gowda M, Kolb J et al (1999) A randomized, controlled trial of the effects of remote, intercessory prayer on outcomes in patients admitted to the coronary care unit. Archives of Internal Medicine 159(19): 2277–8.

30 Bernardi L, Sleight P, Bandinelli G, Wdowczyc-Szulc J (2001) Effect of rosary prayer and yoga mantras on autonomic cardiovascular rhythms: comparative study. British Medical Journal 323: 1446–9.

31 Maltby J, Lewis C, Day L (1999) Religious orientation and psychological well-
    being: The role of the frequency of personal prayer. British Journal of Health
    Psychology 4: 363–78.
32 Wilkinson P (1999) A prayer a day keeps the blues away. The Times. Friday, 12
    November, p 5.
33 Manning M (1994) Healing hands. Kindred Spirit 3(2): 26–8.
34 Petty J (2002) personal communication.
35 McKay B, Musil L (1999) The spiritual healing project. Oxford: De Numine,
    the Newsletter of the Alistair Hardy Society. September. No. 27, pp 11–27.
36 Leibovici L (2001) Effects of remote, retroactive intercessory prayer on out-
    come in patients with bloodstream infection: randomised controlled trial.
    British Medical Journal 323: 1450–1.
37 Rees W, Low-Beer T, Dover S (1987) Terminal cancer patients referred for hos-
    pice care who were not terminally ill and did not have cancer. British Medical
    Journal 295: 318.

Chapter 9 How is Healing Achieved?

1   Hawkes N (2002) One last effort may rid the world of polio. The Times.
    Wednesday, 17 April, p 13.
2   Zaehner R (1959) A New Buddha and a New Tao. In RC Zaehner (Ed) Living
    Faiths. London. Hutchinson, pp 409–10.
3   Lavan S, Williams G (1986) The Unitarian and Universalist Traditions. In RL
    Numbers and D Amundsen (Eds) Caring and Curing: Health and Medicine in
    the Western Religious Traditions. Baltimore: Johns Hopkins University Press,
    p 366.
4   Craze R (1998) with John T'ieh Fou. Traditional Chinese Medicine. London:
    Teach YourselfBooks/Hodder and Stoughton, p 102.
5   Ostrander S, Schroeder L (1971) Psychic Discoveries behind the Iron Curtain.
    London: Bantam Books, p 164.
6   Green B (2000) The Elegant Universe. London: Vintage, p 6.
7   New English Bible. Luke 8: 45–6.
8   Angelo J and Angelo J (2001) Sacred Healing. London: Piatkus, p 80.
9   Psalms 46: 10. King James Version.
10 Govinda Lama A (1960) Foundation of Tibetan Mysticism. London: Rider, p
    158.
11 Govinda Lama A (1977) Creative Meditation and Multidimensional
    Consciousness. London: Unwin, Mandala Edition, pp 54–5.
12 Scrivener J (2000) Personal communication.
13 Boyd H (2000) No stone upturned. Sainsbury magazine. December, pp 206–7.
14 Raphael K (1987) Crystal Healing. The Therapeutic Application of Crystals
    and Stones. Volume. 2. Santa Fe: Aurora Press, p 14.
15 Hurley J, Saunders H (1932) Aquarian Age Healing. USA: Haynes
    Corporation. Facsimile copy published 1999 by Society of Metaphysicians,
    Hastings, Sussex.

16 Stubbs E (1986) Hands and Healing. Friends Fellowship of Healing. Pamphlet 6, pp 5–6.
17 Ryeland J (1999) Newsletter: Summer. London: The Christian Healing Mission, p 4.
18 Jones P (1999) Brochure issued by Cautley House.
19 Ashton P (1993) The Principles and Practice of Christian Healing. In Y Weinidogaeth Iachâu: The Ministry of Healing, Wales. Eglwys Bresbyteraidd Cymru: The Presbyterian Church in Wales, p 24.

Chapter 10 Healing by Deliverance

1 Bishop of Exeter's Commission (1964) Exorcism. Dom Robert Petitpierre (Ed) (1972) London: SPCK.
2 Archbishop of York Study Group (1974) The Christian Ministry of Healing and Deliverance: York.
3 Christian Deliverance Study Group (1996) Deliverance, Psychic Deliverance and Occult Involvement. Michael Perry (Ed) London: SPCK.
4 A Report for the House of Bishops on the Ministry of Healing (2000) A Time to Heal. London: Church House Publishing.
5 General Synod of the Church of England (1975) Report of Proceedings. vol. 6, no. 2.
6 Lewis D (1989) Healing: Fiction, Fantasy or Fact? London: Hodder and Stoughton, pp 122–4.
7 Richards J (1990) Exorcism, Deliverance and Healing. Some Pastoral and Liturgical Guidelines. Cambridge: Grove Books, p 12.
8 Spae J (1972) Shinto Man. Tokyo: Oriens Institute for Religious Research, pp 36–9.
9 Raphael K (1987) Crystal Healing. The Therapeutic Application of Crystals and Stones. Volume 11. Santa Fe: Aurora Press, pp 75–7.
10 Richards J (1990) Exorcism, Deliverance and Healing. Some Pastoral and Liturgical Guidelines. Cambridge: Grove Books, pp 19–21.
11 Christian Deliverance Study Group (1996) Deliverance, Psychic Deliverance and Occult Involvement. Michael Perry (Ed) London: SPCK, pp 133–4.
12 Richards J (1990) Exorcism, Deliverance and Healing. Some Pastoral and Liturgical Guidelines. Cambridge: Grove Books, p 16.
13 BBC2 (2002) The Exorcist. Wednesday, 16 January.
14 The New English Bible (1970) Genesis 3: 1 and 14.
15 Lewis D (1989) Healing: Fiction, Fantasy or Fact? London: Hodder and Stoughton, p 124.
16 The New English Bible (1970) Matthew 11: 18.
17 The New English Bible (1970) Luke 11: 14–19.
18 O'Connor J (2002) A memorable patient. Ernest. British Medical Journal 325: 773.
19 Edgington K (2002) A memorable patient: The devil in detail. British Medical Journal 324: 108.

20 Fisher E (2000) Catholics and Jews confront the Holocaust and each other. World Faiths Encounter No 16, July, 3–13.

21 Weisel E (1982) Night. London: Bantam Books, pp 32 and 64.

22 Weisel E (1982) Night. London: Bantam Books.

23 Lewis D (1989) Healing: Fiction, Fantasy or Fact? London: Hodder and Stoughton, p 340.

24 Christian Deliverance Study Group (1996) Deliverance. Psychic Deliverance and Occult Involvement. Michael Perry (Ed). London: SPCK.

25 Rees W (1971) The hallucinations of widowhood. British Medical Journal 4: 37–41.

26 Silverman P, Worden J (1993) Children's reactions to the death of a parent. In Margaret S Stroebe, Wolfgang Stroebe and Robert O Hanson (Eds) Handbook of Bereavement. Cambridge: Cambridge University Press. pp 300–16.

27 Willis T (2002) Personal communication.

28 Coggan D (1989) Cuthbert Bardsley. Bishop-Evangelist-Pastor. London: Collins, pp 212–13.

29 Francis L, Robbins M, Kay W (2000) Pastoral Care Today: Practice, Problems and Priorities in Churches Today. Published by CWR, Waverley Abbey House, Farnham, Surrey, p 9.

30 Francis L, Robbins M, Kay W (2000) Pastoral Care Today: Practice, Problems and Priorities in Churches Today. Published by CWR, Waverley Abbey House, Farnham, Surrey, pp 20–29.

31 Lewis D (1989) Healing: Fiction, Fantasy or Fact? London: Hodder and Stoughton, pp 339–41.

32 Lewis D (1989) Healing: Fiction, Fantasy or Fact? London: Hodder and Stoughton, p 346 and Whimber J (1985) Power Evangelism. Hodder and Stoughton, pp 44–46.

33 Lewis D (1989) Healing: Fiction, Fantasy or Fact? London: Hodder and Stoughton, p 136.

34 Lewis D (1989) Healing: Fiction, Fantasy or Fact? London: Hodder and Stoughton, p 136.

35 Clark M (1989) Nevra in a Greek village: metaphor, symptom, or disorder? Health Care Women International 10 (2–3): 195–218.

36 Pfeifer S (1994) Belief in demons and exorcism in psychiatric patients in Switzerland. British Journal of Medical Psychology 67(3): 247–58.

37 Amuyunzu M (1998) Willing the spirits to reveal themselves: rural Kenyan mothers' responsibility to restore their children's health. Medical Anthropology Quarterly 12 (4): 490–502.

38 Desai S (2002) personal communication.

39 Parsons S (2000) Ungodly Fear. Fundamentalist Christianity and the Abuse of Power. Oxford: Lion Publishing.

Chapter 11 The Drawbacks of Healing

1 Basynat B (2002) Personal view of Pilgrimage medicine. British Medical Journal 324: 745.

2   Ernst E, White A (2000) Acupuncture may be associated with serious side effects. British Medical Journal 320: 513–14.

3   Ernst E (2000) Risks associated with complementary therapies. In MNG Dukes and JK Aronson (Eds) Meyler's Side Effects of Drugs (fourteenth edition). Amersterdam: Elsevier Science B.V., pp 1469–81.

4   Farah M, Edwards P, Lindquist M, Leon C (2000) International monitoring of adverse health effects associated with herbal medicines. Pharmaco-epidemiology and Drug Safety 9: 105–12.

5   Leon C (2000) personal communication.

6   Periharic L, Shaw D, Colbridge M, House I, Leon C, Murray V (1994) Toxocological problems resulting from exposure to traditional remedies and food supplements. 11(4): 284–94.

7   Nortier J et al (2000) Urolethial carcinoma associated with the use of a Chinese herb (Aristolochia fangchi). The New England Journal of Medicine 342: 1686–7.

8   Periharic L, Shaw D, Leon C, De Smet P, Murray V (1995) Possible association of liver damage with the use of Chinese herbal medicines for skin disease. Vet Human Toxicology 37(6): 583–6.

9   Gould M (2001) Patients warned of dangers of Chinese medicines, British Medical Journal (News.) 323: 720.

10 Metcalfe K, Corns C, Fahie-Wilson M, Mackenzie P (2002) Chinese medicines for slimming will cause health problems. British Medical Journal (Letters) 324: 679.

11 Parsons S (2000) Ungodly Fear: Fundamentalist Christianity and the Abuse of Power. Oxford: Lion Publishing.

12 Woodhouse D (2000) Healing the abused. Acorn. The Magazine of the Acorn Christian Foundation. Issue 6. Spring, p 7.

13 Rome (2002) Vatican says new rules don't bar gay priests. The Tablet. 16 November, p 30.

14 Woodhouse, D (2000) Healing the abused. Acorn. The Magazine of the Acorn Christian Foundation. Issue 6. Spring.

15 Gunston J (1986) We Believe in Healing. Dr Ann England (Ed). East Sussex: Highland Books, p 156.

16 Petticrew M, Bell R, Hunter D (2000) Influence of psychological coping on survival and recurrence in people with cancer: systematic review. British Medical Journal 325: 1066–9.

17 Parsons, S (2000)Ungodly Fear. Fundamentalist Christianity and the Abuse of Power. Oxford: Lion Publishing, pp 17–18.

18 House of Bishops of the General Synod of the Church of England (2000) A Time to Heal. London: Church House Publishing, p xiii.

Chapter 12 Does it Work?

1   Loudon I (1992) The transformation of maternal mortality. British Medical Journal 305: 1557–60.

2   United Nations (1997) Department of Economic and Social Affairs. Statistics Division. Statistical Year-book (42nd issue). Geneva.

3   BBC (2000) Survey commissioned by the BBC and quoted in the Report by a
    Select Committee of the House of Lords on Complementary and Alternative
    Medicine (2000) London: The Stationery Office, p 15.
4   Rees W (1968) Personal view. British Medical Journal 1: 701.
5   National Federation of Spiritual Healers (2002) What is Spiritual Healing?
    Leaflet. Sunbury-on-Thames.
6   English D (1999) Quoted by Esmond Jeffries in The Vision of the Risen Christ.
    Life-Line Issue No. 31, February. The Newsletter of the Pin Mill Christian
    Healing Fellowship. Felixstowe, Suffolk.
7   Rees W, Lutkins S (1967) Mortality of bereavement. British Medical Journal 4:
    13–16.
8   Shakespeare W (1603) Hamlet. I. v. 166.

Index